OXFORD MEDICAL PUBLICATIONS

The economics of
health in developing countries

The economics of
health in developing countries

Edited by

KENNETH LEE

Nuffield Centre for Health Services Studies,
University of Leeds

and

ANNE MILLS

Evaluation and Planning Centre,
London School of Hygiene and Tropical Medicine,
University of London

OXFORD NEW YORK TORONTO
OXFORD UNIVERSITY PRESS
1983

Oxford University Press, Walton Street, Oxford OX2 6DP

London Glasgow New York Toronto
Delhi Bombay Calcutta Madras Karachi
Kuala Lumpur Singapore Hong Kong Tokyo
Nairobi Dar es Salaam Cape Town
Melbourne Auckland

and associated companies in
Beirut Berlin Ibadan Mexico City Nicosia

OXFORD is a trade mark of Oxford University Press

British Library Cataloguing in Publication Data

The Economics of health in developing countries.
1. Underdeveloped areas—Medical care
2. Underdeveloped areas—Medical economics
I. Lee, Kenneth, 1944-   II. Mills, Anne
338.4'73621'091724   RA394
ISBN 0-19-261385-5

Library of Congress Cataloging in Publication Data

Main entry under title:
The Economics of health in developing countries.
(Oxford medical publications)
Bibliography: p.
Includes index.
Contents: Developing countries, health and health
economics / Kenneth Lee and Anne Mills—Economic
development, health services, and health / George
Cumper—Health sector financing and expenditure
surveys / Adrian Mills—[etc.]
    1. Underdeveloped areas—Medical economics.
I. Lee, Kenneth, 1944-   II. Mills, Anne.
III. Series.
RA410.5.E26   1983   338.4'73621'091724   82-22593
ISBN 0-19-261385-5

Typeset by Joshua Associates, Oxford.
Printed in Hong Kong

Preface

We have commissioned in this book a selection of essays which cover as comprehensively as possible, within a single volume, a range of important macro and micro economic issues that economists, planners, policy-makers, professionals, and others face in the health sector. All the contributors to this volume have direct knowledge and experience of working in developing countries, whether for governments, educational institutions, or international agencies. They were asked to choose an area which reflected their particular interests and expertise, and to produce a chapter which would show the reader as clearly as possible the uses of applying economic theories, concepts, and techniques to the health issues of developing countries, and also the technical difficulties they face in so doing. In total, a dozen economists collaborated and eleven chapters were the result.

Each chapter is a review of the 'state of the art' in a particular area, and includes theoretical developments, methods, and techniques, and empirical findings. As editors, we have required each contributor to attempt to clarify the relation between economic theory and real world problems by making full use of their own experiences. Economic theory after all is meant to be about the real world. As for the actual choice of health issues and economic approaches, this is inevitably idiosyncratic: our criteria were that the health policy issues selected should be of current significance; they should draw on a number of theoretical aspects of economics; and they should in all cases combine economic theory and applied economics.

This volume originated in our concern—as economists, teachers, researchers, and advisers—about the lack of suitable texts in this field of study. The economics of health is undoubtedly a rapidly expanding area of academic interest and a focus of local, national, and international attention; yet very few publications have appeared on the economics of the health sector in developing countries. In this volume, intended to help overcome this shortage, we aim to provide a relatively non-technical analysis of the issues for a general and international audience of health practitioners, politicians, academics, and students of health and health care. We expect that the work will be of interest to both fellow economists and prospective economists, but our prime concern throughout has been to keep professional as well as academic needs in mind.

On the subject of acknowledgements, we are indebted to the contributors who have, by their efforts, made this volume possible. The views and interpretations belong to the authors, and do not necessarily represent the views of fellow contributors, international organizations, or the institutions for which they have worked or are working. Both individually and collectively, we are indebted to all the people with whom we have been in regular contact during the course of our work on the economics of health in developing countries. Many people in many countries have given generously of their time and their ideas, and we are most grateful.

One person must be singled out, and we do so with profound gratitude. Jane Thompson has seen the development of this book from the very first ideas to the finished manuscript. Despite our frequent absences abroad, and undeterred by her previous experience of our methods of composition and editing, she has managed with unlimited patient care to prepare this volume for publication.

Leeds and London   K. L.
August 1982   A. M.

Contents

Contributors

Andrew Creese is a Lecturer in Development Studies in the Centre for Development Studies, University College Swansea. After postgraduate work at the London School of Economics, he spent two years in Malawi with the British Council. Following further postgraduate work at Oxford University, he was jointly appointed Lecturer in Health Economics at St. Thomas's Hospital Medical School and the London School of Economics. He has carried out research and published on economic aspects of short-stay surgery, home versus hospital care for the disabled, and resource allocation principles in the English National Health Service. He joined the Institute of Development Studies (Sussex) Ghana Health Project on secondment in 1976-77, and subsequently the Centre for Development Studies in 1978. He has undertaken assignments for the World Health Organization in the Philippines, Indonesia, Thailand, and Brazil, and for the World Bank. He is author of several articles on health economics in both a UK and developing country context.

George Cumper is a Senior Lecturer in Health Economics in the Evaluation and Planning Centre, Ross Institute, London School of Hygiene and Tropical Medicine. He graduated from the University of Cambridge and in 1949 joined the staff of the Institute of Social and Economic Research, University of the West Indies, where he was Professor of Economics from 1966 to 1972. He has written extensively on Caribbean development problems. From 1972 to 1974 and 1976 to 1979 he worked with the South-East Asia Regional Office of the World Health Organization, taking part in national health planning work in Nepal, Thailand, Burma, Bangladesh, and Sri Lanka. More recently he has acted as a consultant for the UK Overseas Development Administration and the World Bank in India and Jamaica. He is editor of *The economy of the West Indies* (1960).

Geoffrey Ferster is a health economist in the Bureau of Health Planning, Ministry of Health, Republic of Indonesia. His doctorate degree is from Cornell University. He has worked on University-based field research in agriculture and community development in Tanzania; and while at the University of Exeter had considerable research experience in health economics and policy planning issues in the National Health Service, including obstetric care, dental health, mental handicap, health care costs, and management information systems. His main areas of responsibility in Indonesia include national long- and medium-term strategic plan formulation, health sector financing and evaluation. He has also advised the World Bank on health financing and project development. He has published widely on these subjects in international journals including *The Lancet* and the *International Journal of Health Services*, and as a contributor to the books prepared by the Nuffield Provincial Hospitals Trust.

Adrian Griffiths is Head of Health Management and Economics at the Sandoz Institute for Health and Socio-Economic Studies, Geneva, and teaches at the Institute of Preventive and Social Medicine, University of Geneva. He trained in economics and then in sociology and social administration at the University of Wales, and before taking up his present post was on the faculty of the Department of Community Health at the London School of Hygiene and Tropical Medicine. His current research includes projects on health sector spending and financing, planning of health services, health service and hospital management, health and related services for the elderly, health information systems, economic evaluation of screening and of medical technology, and use of clinical resources. He has served as a consultant to the World Health Organization, the Organization for Economic Co-operation and Development, and the Council of Europe. He is the author and co-editor of numerous scientific papers, reports, and books including *Economics and health policy* (1980), *An annotated bibliography of health economics, Western European sources* (1980), and *Health sector financing and expenditure: manual of survey methodology for developing countries* (1982).

Kenneth Lee is a Lecturer in Health Economics at the Nuffield Centre for Health Services Studies, University of Leeds, and also holds Associate appointments in the School of Economic Studies and the Department of Social Policy and Administration. He graduated from the University of Hull, and undertook postgraduate work at the Universities of Leicester and Keele. He has carried out research and written extensively on approaches to health economics, health planning and management, care of the elderly, primary health care, and emergency health services; and undertaken assignments on behalf of the World Health Organization in Europe, South-East Asia, and the Western Pacific. He is co-editor of *NHS reorganisation: issues and prospects* (1974) and *Conflicts in the National Health Service* (1977); editor of *Economics and health planning* (1979); and co-author (with Anne Mills) of *Policy-making and planning in the health Sector* (1982).

Anne Mills is a lecturer in Health Economics in the Evaluation and Planning Centre, Ross Institute, London School of Hygiene and Tropical Medicine, and also part-time Lecturer at the Nuffield Centre for Health Services Studies, University of Leeds. She graduated from the University of Oxford, and then went to Malawi as an Overseas Development Institute Fellow to work as the economist in the Ministry of Health. After postgraduate work in health economics at the

Nuffield Centre, she joined the staff to do research on strategic and annual planning in the National Health Service. She now works in a multi-disciplinary unit focusing on the evaluation of health-related services in developing countries, and her activities have included work for the World Health Organization in Thailand and Geneva, and for the British Government in West Africa, the Caribbean and Middle East. She is author of a number of articles on issues of health planning and health economics, and of *Policy-making and planning in the health sector* (with Kenneth Lee).

Michael Mills is an economist presently working in the Population, Health, and Nutrition Department of the World Bank. He graduated from the University of Cambridge, and undertook postgraduate work at the Universities of Sussex and Leicester. After carrying out a research project for the Department of Health and Social Security, he went to Botswana as an Overseas Development Institute Fellow. There he worked first in the Ministry of Finance and Development Planning, and then in the Ministry of Health. After completion of his ODI Fellowship, he continued to work in Botswana under the British Government's aid programme, and has subsequently undertaken assignments on behalf of the Commonwealth Secretariat in Zimbabwe, and the World Bank in Thailand. He is co-author of *Health sector financing and expenditure: manual of survey methodology for developing countries* (with Adrian Griffiths).

Nicholas Prescott is a graduate of Oxford University and presently works as a consultant to the Policy and Research Unit of the Population, Health, and Nutrition Department, The World Bank. He has served previously as a consultant to the World Health Organization and the Asian Development Bank. Publications include a co-edited *Annotated bibliography of health economics: Western European Sources* (1980), and a number of papers on health economics in developing and developed countries.

Robert Tilden has been working in the International Health area for the last eleven years, and is presently employed with the Indonesian Ministry of Health as a consultant to its Vitamin A Deficiency Prevention Programme. Previously he worked with the Sarawak, East Malaysia Ministry of Health in developing its Rural Health Improvement Scheme. His graduate studies have taken place at the University of Michigan, and he is presently a non-resident Lecturer for the Department of Health Planning and Administration, School of Public Health, in the same University. His publications have appeared in a number of journals including the *Bulletin of the World Health Organization*, the *American Journal of Clinical Nutrition, Proceedings of the Third Asian Nutrition Conference,* and the *American Journal of Public Health.*

Jeremy Warford is Chief, Policy and Research Unit of the Population, Health, and Nutrition Department of the World Bank. He has a Bachelor's degree in

Economics and Government from the University of Bristol and a Ph.D. in Economics from the University of Manchester. After postgraduate work he taught at the University of Manchester, then became Research Associate at the Brookings Institution, Washington DC. He joined the World Bank in 1970, and became Economic Adviser to the Energy, Water, and Telecommunications Department. In early 1979, he joined the Asian Development Bank, Manila, where he was Deputy Director, Infrastructure Department; he returned to the World Bank in October 1980, where he assumed his current position. He has worked in many developing countries, and published several articles and books; he is author of *Public policy toward general aviation* (1971); and co-author of *Village water supply: economics and policy in the developing world* (1976), and *Electricity pricing: theory and case studies* (1982).

Gill Westcott is a Lecturer in Development Economics at the Nuffield Centre for Health Services Studies, University of Leeds. She received her training in economics at the Universities of Cambridge and Oxford, and her graduate studies involved field work in India on agricultural extension programmes. She then worked for five years in South Africa, at a hospital in the Transkei and at the University of Cape Town, researching into health problems and their socio-economic background, including the utilization of primary health care facilities, agricultural practices, child malnutrition, and family incomes in rural areas. At the Nuffield Centre she teaches health economics, development economics and social policy, and is currently researching the impact of unemployment on health in a UK setting.

Mark Wheeler is a Lecturer at the Project Planning Centre for Developing Countries, University of Bradford. He graduated from the University of Oxford, and did postgraduate work at the London School of Economics. He then worked for several years in Zambia and Kenya, before returning to the Medical Care Research Unit at the London School of Hygiene and Tropical Medicine to undertake research on the British National Health Service. Before taking up his present post, he was Senior Planning Officer in the Malawi Ministry of Health. He has written various articles on health manpower and health services planning, and has served as a consultant for the World Health Organization and the UK Overseas Development Administration in Indonesia, Cameroon, the Seychelles, and the Solomon Islands.

Tables

Figures

1

Developing countries, health, and health economics

Kenneth Lee and Anne Mills

Introduction

All citizens share an interest in health and health care, and it is in the national interest that the resources available for health should be spent effectively. Regardless of their stage of development or level of income, people desire an improvement in their state of health, greater access to a wide range of health and health-related services, and to enjoy the benefits of scientific and technological advances that will assist these aims. Their governments share these objectives, but in managing the economy must allocate limited resources between competing uses and decide which popular demands to satisfy.

These features are common to all countries, but it is useful to make a broad distinction between those countries classed as 'developed' and those classed as 'developing'. Developed countries have far better standards of living, far higher levels of health, extensive and highly sophisticated health services, and the ability and resources to develop, if they so wish, yet more sophisticated health technologies. In developing countries, many millions of people are desperately poor, experience high levels of mortality, morbidity, and disability and have little or no access to modern health services.

While a contrast can be drawn between the circumstances of developing and developed countries, developing countries themselves are by no means a homogeneous group. They include the small nation states of the Caribbean, the huge countries of India and China, some rapidly industrializing countries such as Korea and Singapore, and the countries ravaged by war and famine such as Kampuchea and parts of the Horn of Africa.

Nevertheless, for the purpose of examining the economics of health, developing countries do have sufficient characteristics in common for them to be classed together (Todaro 1977). Their common characteristics, visible in their economies, their morbidity and mortality experience, and their disease patterns, are explored in the first part of this chapter in order to provide the context for subsequent chapters. The discipline of economics is then introduced and health economics is put in historical perspective to indicate the nature of its concerns and to justify its relevance to thehealth sector in developing countries. Finally, the chapter summarizes the scope of this book, indicating the aspects

TABLE 1.1. *Economic indicators of selected countries*

Selected countries by GNP per capita	GNP per capita		Adult literacy rate (%) 1976*	% labour force in		Urban population	
	($) 1979	Average annual growth rate (%) 1960–79		Agriculture 1979	Industry 1979	% of total population 1980	Average annual growth rate (%) 1970–80
UK	6320	2.2	99	2	42	91	0.3
US	10 630	2.4	99	2	32	73	1.5
Industrial market economies	9440	4.0	99	6	38	77	1.3
Brazil	1780	4.8	76	40	22	65	3.7
Nigeria	670	3.7	N/A	55	18	20	4.7
Thailand	590	4.6	84	77	9	14	3.3
Bolivia	550	2.2	63	50	24	33	4.1
Yemen Arab Republic	420	10.9	13	76	11	10	7.2
Kenya	380	2.7	45	78	10	14	6.8
Middle income countries	1420	3.8	72	43	23	50	3.8
Indonesia	370	4.1	62	59	12	20	4.0
Zaïre	260	0.7	15	75	13	34	7.2
Sri Lanka	230	2.2	85	54	14	27	3.6
Malawi	200	2.9	25	86	5	10	6.8
India	190	1.4	36	71	11	22	3.3
Ethiopia	130	1.3	15	80	7	15	6.6
Low income countries	230	1.6	51	71	14	17	3.7

N/A = Not available
*Rates refer to a variety of years, generally not more than two years different from that specified
Source: World Bank 1981a

of health economics that it covers and the sequence of arguments that are to be found within it.

Economic characteristics of developing countries

A variety of labels can be applied to developing countries; they may be called 'developing', 'less-developed', or 'poor' countries, the 'Third World' (in contrast to the First World, economically advanced 'capitalist' countries, and the Second World, 'socialist' countries), and most recently, the 'South' (Brandt Commission 1980). Within this broad classification, countries can be sub-classified in a variety of ways depending on the focus of interest. One of the most frequently used classification schemes is that adopted by the World Bank which ranks countries by per capita Gross National Product (GNP) (World Bank 1981*a*). 'Low-income' countries are those with a national income per capita of $370 or less in 1979, and 'middle-income' countries those with 1979 per capita income of more than $370 which are still recognizable as 'developing'. Within this grouping of developing countries, a distinction is made between those which are oil exporters and those which import oil, since this factor is a crucial influence on their current economic progress and future prospects.

The distinction between low and middle income emphasizes perhaps the major characteristic of developing countries, namely low levels of income and therefore low standards of living. Table 1.1 shows the (weighted) average per capita incomes calculated by the World Bank for low-income, middle-income, and industrial market countries (with a population of one million or more). Thirty-six low-income countries had an average per capita income in 1979 of $230; 62 middle-income countries a per capita income of $1420; and 18 industrial market economies a per capita income of $9440 (World Bank 1981*a*). Such a comparison throws into stark relief the differences between the developed and the developing world. Moreover, as Table 1.1 also indicates, richer countries have in general experienced higher growth rates in per capita income than poorer countries. Thus the income gap between rich and poor has been widening, not narrowing.

Any change in per capita income over time reflects two influences, the rate of growth of GNP and the rate of growth of population. The widening gap between rich and poor countries has resulted not only from relatively slower economic growth in poor countries, but also from their high population growth rates which have meant that the benefits of any economic growth have had to be spread over more people. Table 1.2 shows that between 1950 and 1980 real per capita incomes rose by less than one-half in low-income countries, and by about two-and-a-half times in middle-income and industrial countries. Indeed, some middle-income countries, the 'newly industrializing' countries such as Korea and Taiwan, have experienced extremely high rates of economic growth.

Such comparisons, which involve converting the Gross Domestic Product (GDP) of each country into US dollars at the prevailing exchange rate, clearly do not necessarily reflect the purchasing power of countries since many goods and services, such as housing, education, and health services, are not internationally

TABLE 1.2. *Growth in income per person 1950-1980*

GNP per person ($) (1980)	1950	1960	1980
Industrial countries	4130	5580	10 660
Middle-income countries	640	820	1580
Low-income countries	170	180	250

Source: World Bank 1981*a*

traded and are often cheaper (relative to traded goods whose prices are reflected in exchange rates) in poor countries. 'Purchasing power parities', which attempt to reflect countries' ability to purchase goods and services, have been calculated for a number of countries and their implications for comparisons of national income per capita are shown in Table 1.3. The difference between rich and poor countries is much reduced in absolute terms, but in relative terms, a marked contrast remains.

TABLE 1.3. *Comparisons of real income, 1980*

Country group	Exchange rate conversion ($)	Purchasing power conversion ($)
Oil importers	790	1700
Low-income	220	730
Middle-income	1710	2690
Oil exporters	1060	2080
All developing countries	850	1790
Industrial countries	10 660	8960

Source: World Bank 1981*a*

The use of GNP as an indicator of standard of living is also unsatisfactory (Seers 1969). GNP per capita is none the less highly correlated with such indicators of welfare as nutritional status and literacy rates (World Bank 1980*a*), and is therefore a rough indicator of welfare itself. Yet it is also a highly aggregate measure. To establish the conditions under which most people live, it is necessary to look at the distribution of national income within countries. Such distribution is often highly unequal: some regions are better off than others; urban dwellers are generally better-off than rural dwellers; and the benefits of development often accrue to only a small portion of the population, those in the modernized industrial and agricultural sectors, while the rural poor remain largely unaffected (Streeten 1979).

Statistics on the extent of poverty are very uncertain. The World Bank estimates that about 750 million people, or almost 40 per cent of the population of the 'South' (Brandt Commission 1980), live in absolute poverty, their income inadequate to obtain even the basic necessities of life. Such poverty is concentrated in sub-Saharan Africa and South Asia, though many better-off countries have areas of acute poverty. On the basis of favourable assumptions about economic growth, the World Bank has estimated that about 630 million will still be in poverty in the year 2000; they could number 750 million if it is assumed that economic prospects are bleak.

What are the economic characteristics that lie behind this picture of low incomes and unequal distribution? Reference should again be made to Table 1.1, which lists some economic indicators for a number of developing countries as well as statistics for the UK and US to provide a basis for comparison. In the first place, the majority of people in developing countries, and the great majority in low-income countries, live and work in rural areas. In Malawi, for example, one of the least developed countries, 86 per cent of the labour force works in agriculture and only 5 per cent in industry. Such figures can be contrasted with 2 per cent and 42 per cent in the United Kingdom.

A second characteristic is that the productivity of agriculture is generally very low: most agriculture is subsistence farming, characterized by primitive technologies, poor organisation, and limited physical and human capital inputs. Despite such low productivity, a significant proportion of national product is generated in agriculture, because that is where the majority of the population work. The characteristic of low levels of human capital is emphasized by statistics on literacy rates. On average, only 51 per cent of adults are literate in low income countries (43 per cent if China and India are excluded), and some of the poorest countries have rates of 20 per cent or less. In contrast, higher education has often expanded too rapidly, leading to unemployment amongst secondary school and university graduates.

Indeed, unemployment or underemployment constitutes a fourth characteristic of developing countries. Open unemployment is generally an urban phenomenon, but in addition, there are many people in rural areas who are underemployed, that is working less than they would like to work. Moreover, employment prospects are not good since the potential labour force is expanding rapidly as a result of high population growth rates. Such problems are particularly acute in the countries of Asia which have a high proportion of landless people.

A further characteristic is historically low but now rapidly increasing rates of urbanization. Low income countries have a minority of their populations living in urban areas, but are experiencing rapid rural–urban migration as rural dwellers attempt to improve their standard of living and that of their families by seeking employment in urban areas. In some countries, the rate and pattern of urbanization is seen by governments as one of their most serious social problems.

Finally, the great majority of developing countries are situated in tropical or semi-tropical areas. This affects their economy in a number of ways: a hot climate reduces the efficiency of labour; land erosion is a more serious problem; climatic conditions encourage the persistence of tropical diseases affecting man, animals, and crops; and most scientific and technological research is directed to solving agricultural and medical problems in temperate climates (Streeten 1979).

In summary, the characteristics common to economies of developing countries include low levels of income and widespread poverty, unequal distribution of income and wealth, a large rural population, a relatively small industrial sector, low levels of productivity stemming from low levels of physical and human capital, high unemployment and underemployment, rapid urbanization, and often difficult climatic and topographical conditions. While developing countries as a group display these characteristics, the extent to which each is evident in a particular developing country varies widely. Some middle-income countries have experienced rapid economic growth, yet the prospects for improved standards of living in the poorest and least-developed countries are not good in the immediate future. Not only has the gap between rich and poor been widening, but so has the gap between the very poor and the less poor.

Aspects of health in developing countries

The economic characteristics of developing countries are reflected in their health characteristics. Per capita income, for example, is highly correlated with indicators such as life expectancy and infant mortality, not only between but also within countries. Table 1.4 lists some of these major health-related indicators for a number of developing countries and for groups of countries classified by their income level.

A striking feature of virtually all developing countries is their high rate of population growth. Very few of the low-income and poorer middle-income countries have had population growth rates over the last ten years of less than 2 per cent per annum. In consequence, a large proportion of their populations are children who will require food, education, and health services before they can become economically productive. Direct health consequences of rapid population growth can include a higher incidence of communicable diseases as a result of overcrowded and poor housing, high maternal mortality and morbidity, and poor nutrition.

Such population growth rates are the product of high fertility and declining death rates. As Table 1.5 indicates, there has been considerable improvement

TABLE 1.5. *Change in life expectancy 1950-1979*

Life expectancy at birth	1950	1960	1979	Increase 1950-79
Industrial countries	67	70	74	7
Middle-income countries	48	53	61	13
Low-income countries	37	42	51	14

Source: World Bank 1981*a*

over the last thirty years in life expectancy rates, though this trend is now slowing (World Bank 1980*b*). The lower life expectancy rates in developing countries are largely attributable to infant and child mortality rates which are many times higher than those in developed countries. In other words, the burden of illness and death in the developing world falls most heavily on babies and small children (see Table 1.6). Moreover, countrywide infant death rates disguise large differences

TABLE 1.4. Health-related indicators

Selected countries by GNP per capita	Average annual growth of population (%) 1970–79	Life expectancy at birth (years) 1979	Infant mortality rate* 1978	Child death rate 1979	Daily per capita calorie supply (% of need) 1977	% of population with access to safe water 1975	Population per Physician 1977*	Population per Nursing person 1977*	Central govt. per capita expenditure on health (1975 $) 1978
UK	0.1	73	14	1	132	N/A	750	300	N/A
US	1.0	74	14	1	135	N/A	570	150	179
Industrial market economies	0.7	74	13	1	131	N/A	620	220	229
Brazil	2.2	63	92	8	107	77	1700	N/A	20†
Nigeria	2.5	49	N/A	22	83	N/A	15 740	4030	2†
Thailand	2.4	62	68	6	105	22	8150	3540	3
Bolivia	2.5	50	N/A	23	83	38	1850	3070	5
Yemen Arab Republic	1.8	42	N/A	41	91	4	12 460	5660	2
Kenya	3.4	55	91	15	88	17	11 630	1090	5
Middle income countries	2.4	61	N/A	10	109	58	4380	1820	15
Indonesia	2.3	53	120	14	105	12	13 640	8850	N/A
Zaïre	2.7	47	N/A	25	104	16	15 530	1940	N/A
Sri Lanka	1.7	66	49	3	96	20	6750	2050	5
Malawi	2.8	47	N/A	25	90	33	40 680	2790	2
India	2.1	52	125	15	91	33	3620	6430	(·)
Ethiopia	2.1	40	N/A	36	75	6	75 320	5400	1†
Low income countries	2.1	57	N/A	17	98	29	16 380‡	14 890‡	2

(·)   Less than half the unit shown
N/A   Not available
*   Rates refer to a variety of years, generally not more than two years different from that specified
†   Figures are for 1977
‡   Weighted average excludes India and China
Source: World Bank 1981a

TABLE 1.6. *Infant and early childhood mortality rates, 1970–1975*

	Infant mortality rate	Child mortality rate
More developed regions		
Country range	8.3–40.3	0.4–2.0
Less developed regions		
Northern Africa	c.130	c.30
Sub-Saharan Africa	c.200	>30
Asia	c.120–130	>10
Latin America	<100 (probably c.85–90)	c.6

Source: WHO 1981

within countries between regions, between families of different income levels, and between rural and urban areas. In Thailand, for example, infant mortality in 1970 was estimated to vary between 87 per thousand live births for mothers with no schooling living outside municipal areas, and 16 for those with secondary or university schooling in municipal areas (Knodel and Chamratrithirong 1977). In 1974/75, a Thai survey showed that the overall infant mortality rate of 56 disguised regional variations, ranging from 31 in Bangkok, through 49 in the rest of the Central Region, to 96 in the North (NSO 1977).

Once children in developing countries have survived to the age of five, they experience a mortality rate much closer to that of developed countries. They remain exposed, however, to a variety of non-fatal conditions, which cause morbidity, debility, and disability. It is estimated that such illnesses disrupt as much as one-tenth of people's time in most developing countries (World Bank 1980*b*).

The disease pattern which produces this mortality and morbidity is quite different from that of developed countries. Infectious and parasitic diseases represent the most significant health problems, especially for children. Diarrhoeal diseases are commonly a leading cause of death amongst children, and intestinal parasitic diseases, with near 100 per cent infection rates for such parasites as hookworm in some communities, can cause chronic debility. Respiratory diseases, such as tuberculosis and pneumonia, and other airborne diseases such as measles are also major causes of mortality and morbidity.

Vector-borne diseases tend to be less serious as causes of mortality, but are major problems in certain areas. For instance, about 1200 million people live in areas where the transmission of malaria still occurs (World Bank 1980*b*), some 200 million people a year are affected by malaria, and about one million infants and children die (Gilles 1981). Some 500 to 600 million people are exposed to the risk of infection with schistosomiasis (bilharzia) and about 200 million are probably infected (Webbe 1981); and well over 250 million are exposed to infection with filariasis (Duke 1981). Other important vector-borne diseases include onchocerciasis (river-blindness) and trypanosomiasis (sleeping sickness).

The most widespread condition affecting the health of children is not, however, any of the above diseases but malnutrition (WHO 1981). It has been estimated that about 100 million children under five years are suffering from protein-energy malnutrition. In parts of Africa the prevalence is over 20 per cent of children under five for severe, and up to 65 per cent for moderate protein-energy malnutrition. The combination of malnutrition with childhood infectious diseases such as measles and whooping cough produces high case fatality rates.

Such a disease pattern is overwhelmingly the result of poverty. Those aspects of poverty that are particularly important, apart from nutrition, are lack of access to safe water, inadequate sanitation and poor housing, and lack of reasonable quality health services. Many diseases spread through the contamination of food, water, or soil with human waste. In 1975, only 29 per cent of populations in low-income countries, and 58 per cent in middle-income countries, had access to safe water. Statistics on sanitation are scarce, but it is clear that rural populations in low-income countries have minimal provision of facilities for waste disposal.

There are an increasing number of demonstrations that the provision of primary health care can do much to improve health, especially of mothers and children (Gwatkin, Wilcox, and Wray 1980). Yet the health services of most developing countries still concentrate their resources and efforts on hospitals which are not accessible for the majority of the population in rural areas and urban slums. Thus countries like Zaïre and Nigeria have only one doctor per 16 000 people, and few low-income countries have more than one 'nursing person' per 2000 people. While primary health care can improve health *relatively* cheaply, providing complete coverage is still likely to strain the resources of the governments of many low-income countries whose health budgets amount to only $1-2 per capita, and who have large rural and widely scattered populations (World Bank 1981*b*).

This summary of the principal causes of mortality and morbidity and of the pattern of disease experienced particularly by the poorer section of the populations of developing countries provides the context for subsequent chapters. Since the health problems are so great and resources so scarce, it is of great importance that the measures countries take to improve health should be both effective and economical in their resource use, and equitable in their design and impact. This chapter therefore now turns to considering the relevance of health economics to these objectives.

Definitions of economics and health economics.

The nature of health economics is best explained by first defining economics:

the study of how people and society end up choosing, with or without the use of money, to employ scarce productive resources that could have alternative uses, to produce various commodities and distribute them for consumption, now or in the future, among various persons and groups in society. It analyses the costs and benefits of improving patterns of resource allocation. (Samuelson 1976).

Such a definition emphasizes economics as the study of scarcity and choice;

of how to choose the best combination of resources to deliver in-patient care for instance, or how best to allocate a given quantity of resources between alternative ways of improving health. The definition does not restrict economics to any one kind of human activity: it applies to all activities where scarcity and choice exist. Its relevance to the health sectors of developing countries, where resources are extremely scarce, is thus evident.

The above quotation describes 'positive' economics which is concerned with 'what is', 'was', or 'will be', disagreement over positive statements being settled by an appeal to the facts. In addition, there is a body of economics which is 'normative', that is which attempts to determine what 'ought to be', not only what is. Such a process requires value judgements to be made about the norms, or standards, to be applied, and disagreement over normative statements cannot be settled by empirical observation. Positive economics uses theory to explain and predict, whereas normative economics goes beyond explanation and prediction to recommend courses of action that will, in terms of the values adopted, improve the well-being of society. Positive economics is not, however, irrelevant to policy-making, for although it cannot dictate what objectives should be achieved, it can explore the implications of adopting different objectives and different policy options.

'Health' economics can be broadly defined as the application of the theories, concepts, and techniques of economics to the health sector. It is thus concerned with such matters as the allocation of resources between various health-promoting activities; the quantity of resources used in health service delivery; the organization and funding of health service institutions; the efficiency with which resources are allocated and used for health purposes; and the effects of preventive, curative, and rehabilitative health services on individuals and society (Lee and Mills 1979b).

There are a number of other disciplines and professions which are equally interested in such topics, and have a useful and often essential part to play in health sector research and policy analysis. The particular contribution of the economist to the examination of these issues rests on the distinctive method of approach, or concepts and theories, and patterns of thought of economics. The kind of approach characteristically adopted by the economist has been described as:

the desire to specify an unambiguous objective or set of objectives against which to judge and monitor policy; the desire to identify the production function; the recognition of the importance of human behaviour, as well as technology and the natural environment, in the causes, prevention, cure and care of disease.

(Culyer 1981)

The economist's views, of course, will represent only one input to policy-making, and the policy-maker will weigh up views from a variety of sources in making his decisions.

Before proceeding, it is helpful to make three further important distinctions: between the economics of health and that of health services, between forms of economic analysis, and between economists and economics. First, while in the past the label of health economics has on occasion been attached only to the economics of health services, it is now generally accepted that health economics is interested in all health-affecting activities; any indeterminacy of the boundaries of health economics will thus stem from the indeterminacy of the health sector itself. Second, health economics encompasses both economic theory and applied economics, the latter using theory to explain practical problems, and to explore the implications of particular courses of action. While such work can be developed and expounded within the walls of a university, it can also be conducted within less rarified surroundings—in government, health administration offices, or health services. An economist can therefore be employed as a scientist or academic, a health policy analyst or adviser, or as a troubleshooter on the spot (Williams 1980). Finally, while economics is the stock-in-trade of the economist, that is the specialist in economics, it need not necessarily be exclusive to economists. Clinicians, other health workers, and health planners can all apply the principles and lessons of health economics, though they would necessarily require some prior introduction to the discipline.

The development of health economics

Health economics is a product mainly of the last two decades, but has reached the stage of development where some present practitioners already feel able to look back over its historical development and review its achievements (Klarman 1979; Rosenthal 1979; Culyer 1981). It has even received the distinction of being surveyed by a contemporary historian (Fox 1979). The habitual practice of health economists, when justifying their interest in health matters, has been to refer to their forerunners and particularly to Sir William Petty in the seventeenth century and Sir Edwin Chadwick in the nineteenth. British economists are indebted to the recent researches of an American health economist, who has taken the trouble to examine in detail some of the ideas of these two men (Fein 1980). These ideas are particularly relevant to the theme of this book, since they were formulated at a time when England could be considered as 'developing', if the present-day system of classifying economic development is applied in a historical context.

Petty, who lived from 1623 to 1687, was an economist and statistician whose work is remembered by health economists for its attempt to quantify the value of human life. His approach will be a familiar one to economists in developing countries, for his measure of an individual's value was expressed in terms of that person's contribution to national production. This led him to calculate that expenditures which saved lives, for instance by improving medicine or evacuating people from London during a plague epidemic, could be considered a good investment as their benefits exceeded their costs. From these calculations he drew the conclusion that:

it is not in the Interest of the State to leave Phisitians and Patients (as now) to their own shifts (Petty 1676, quoted in Fein 1980).

Similar ideas were advanced by Chadwick (1800–1890), one of the disciples of the English movement known as Benthamites or Utilitarians who influenced public health legislation in the first half of the nineteenth century:

As the artist for his purpose views the human being as a subject for the cultivation of the beautiful—as the physiologist for the cultivation of his art views him solely as a material organism, so the economist for the advancement of his science may well treat the human being simply as an investment of capital, in productive force (Chadwick 1862, again quoted in Fein 1980).

Chadwick argued that better sanitation was a good investment, and that prevention of disease could offer greater benefit than the building of hospitals to treat those diseases.

These ideas have obvious similarities to contemporary ideas on health strategies and on the importance of health improvement in developing countries. Moreover, then as now, it was accepted that the values of politicians and decision-makers should not be narrow financial ones, but that economic arguments could be used to support the moral judgement that the health of populations should be improved.

Such arguments on the productive value of human life, now known as the human capital approach, were not however incorporated into the mainstream of economic theory until the late 1940s and 1950s, though some attempts to apply the approach continued, in particular to assess the economic cost of disease. Prescott (1979) quotes a number of early examples of such studies: an attempt to quantify the number of disability days due to an acute malaria attack and to assess its implications for agricultural output on a plantation in Louisiana, USA (Van Dine 1916); aggregate estimates of the economic effects of malaria in India in terms of lost output resulting from mortality, disability, and debility (Sinton 1935; Sinton 1936); and a detailed survey of five Indian villages to investigate the effect of malaria on labour supply and earnings (Russell and Menon 1942).

Other work related to health economics was going on at this time in developed countries. Much of it was termed medical economics, and included gathering financial and social information on health care utilization patterns, investigating the efficiency of hospitals, exploring the desirability of health insurance, and looking at the business side of medical practice (Fox 1979). However, this had few connections with the discipline of economics, nor did it look to economic theory for help in explaining its observations. Indeed, the growth of health economics as a sub-discipline of economics can be dated only from the 1950s (in the United States) and the 1960s (in the United Kingdom) when a number of professional economists began to apply their concepts and theories to the health field.

Rosenthal (1979) has identified three circumstances which in his view contributed to this growth of interest amongst American economists in health and medical care:

(1) the application of the techniques of economic analysis was proving of considerable assistance to decision-making in federal agencies:
(2) there was increased awareness that the economic resources being devoted to the production and distribution of medical care were both large and increasing; and
(3) the discipline of economics was developing more complex and elaborate theories of human behaviour that were potentially susceptible to empirical testing and refinement.

One result of this increasing interest in developed countries has been the appearance of annotated bibliographies of health economics (Culyer, Wiseman, and Walker 1977; Griffiths, Rigoni, Tacier, and Prescott 1980) and the introduction of academic teaching and research programmes in health economics (Lee and Mills 1979*b*). Another trend has been for more economists to turn their attention to aspects of applied economics such as health planning, management, and clinical behaviour, both by working outside their traditional base of economics departments, in medical schools, government health agencies, and local health authorities; and by promoting the acceptance of economic ideas and techniques amongst other professional groups such as clinicians and health planners, managers, and administrators (Lee and Mills 1979*a*).

While the work being done has had considerable coherence, as the application of economics to health, economists debate amongst themselves whether they should advocate how health services 'ought' to be provided, or restrict themselves to analyses of how the sector works in practice, of alternative ways of allocating scarce resources, and of the implications of different policies: that is to what is and what might be. These differences over role definition manifest themselves most clearly in the division betwen those economists who give priority in their work to the achievement of health sector *efficiency* through an emphasis on the operation of a market for health care and on the benefits of competition, and those who give priority to *equity*, that is to achieving a more equal or fairer distribution of access to health services and health status, if necessary through increased government intervention (Fein 1980). The interested reader will trace such differences of emphasis within the covers of this book.

In developing countries, a recent increase both in the numbers of economists working on health issues and in the literature in this field has been noticeable, though to a lesser extent than in Western Europe and North America. Countries have been attempting to expand their expertise in health economics, if necessary with outside assistance, and have been given encouragement and help by the World Health Organization and the World Bank. International agencies have been recruiting health economists, both for their own purposes and to work on assignments for developing countries. There are also the beginnings of a body of basic health economics literature better suited to the circumstances of developing countries (WHO 1975; Sorkin 1976; Abel-Smith 1976; Griffiths and Bankowski 1980) and of case study material which applies economic concepts and techniques to the health field (Djukanovic and Mach 1975; Abel-Smith and Leiserson 1978; WHO 1978). Developing countries have, as yet, produced few health economists of their own. There are a few working on health issues in academic departments of economics, a few in schools of medicine and health research institutes, and a few working as health planners in ministries of health or development planning. Of the health economists in or from developed countries, only a few work on the health issues of the developing world.

Some features of the work economists have been doing on developing country health issues distinguish it from work done on developed country issues and are worth noting here. First, its links are to development economics as much as to the main body of economics, and this lends it a number of characteristics. For instance, the ideas of development economics have shaped the emphasis of health economics: models of economic growth have in the past emphasized shortage of capital and the need to increase material production, giving second place to expenditure for social purposes such as health. In response, health economics, drawing on its own traditions, emphasized the relationship between improved health and improved output, though without being able to demonstrate this conclusively, except in special circumstances. Recently, ideas on the most appropriate strategies for development have emphasized considerations of income distribution and the targeting of development efforts on those groups in the greatest need (Livingstone 1981). Such ideas have assisted the now general acceptance of health expenditures as justified by their direct contribution to people's welfare, rather than by their indirect contribution via output. Implicit within this new approach is the notion that health improvements are not necessarily dependent on improvements in economic well-being, for instance as measured by per capita GNP (Cumper 1982). Increased emphasis is now placed, therefore, on the scope for re-allocating resources to the health sector, and on increasing the internal efficiency of the health sector, for instance through organizational and social changes and the adoption of different technologies.

This point emphasizes another legacy from development economics, namely a stress on the applied side of the discipline. Health economists have paid particular attention to the needs of practitioners and policy-makers for advice, and a number of economists work not only as academics but also as advisers, planners, and implementors. Indeed, applied health economics has been associated for some time with health planning, for instance via the PAHO/CENDES method of health planning and Country Health Programming, and by health economists working as health planners (Gish 1975; Mills 1975). Rarely has there been more than sporadic involvement in expanding the theoretical body of knowledge.

A second feature of health economics in developing countries stems from their links with international and bilateral agencies, especially those concerned with aid. Health economists are increasingly consulted and employed by international organizations either as internal advisers or to assist recipient countries. This kind of work can pose moral dilemmas for economists. Health economists may also run the risk of being used by aid donors or recipients to provide a façade of respectability to projects formulated and decisions made without regard to economic advice, as development economists have experienced (Giles 1979). Moreover, the dependence of a number of countries on health aid and on imported health products adds an international dimension to health economics and the study of health policy-making.

A final distinctive feature of health economics in developing countries is perhaps not surprising: its concentration on those health issues and problems of paramount concern to such countries. A fairly extensive literature exists, for example, on the economic cost of specific diseases and on the costs of their control or eradication. More recently, economists have become involved in issues of health care financing, primary health care, and appropriate technology. These strategies have obliged economists to look also into the socioeconomic context within which changes to promote health have to be introduced (Cumper 1982), thus requiring them to understand local influences on health behaviour, including cultural factors and the role of traditional medicine as well as social structures and institutional behaviour.

The justification for health economics.

In exploring the historical development of the sub-discipline of health economics, some of the reasons why health economics has become popular amongst governments in developing countries have been mentioned. What justification is there for believing it can become an important and popular field of study in developing countries?

Economic considerations play a key role in all aspects of life: in agriculture, housing, industry, trade, and in health. In addition, the nature and level of a country's economic development can be shown to be a major determinant of its epidemiological profile, and is clearly associated with the level of health service and health-related activities a country can support. Its ideological commitment, economic philosophy, and organizational structures will then shape how much of, and where, such activities are provided. Health policy and its implementation is thus strongly influenced by macroeconomic considerations.

At the same time, the health of a population can itself influence economic progress. Health programmes have therefore come to be seen as part of a comprehensive strategy aimed at improving the social and economic welfare of populations. Such a strategy demands the selection of those programmes which improve health most efficiently: health services, or the provision of other infrastructure such as water and sanitation, or actions aimed at improving nutrition, for instance.

The reappraisal of health policies in a number of developing countries has involved questioning the merits of many existing forms of care, and of past strategies and priorities. Choices on how best to improve health exist everywhere, but such choices in poor countries are both crucial and difficult. Efforts to widen the choices to be considered for delivering health services and for encouraging health-promoting activities are therefore highly relevant.

They are particularly relevant in the economic context of poor countries. Health services absorb a significant proportion of both government expenditure and family budgets. They also demand scarce foreign exchange for drugs, equipment, and transport, and many countries are experiencing escalating medical costs. Governments are actively seeking ways of containing costs and increasing efficiency. Health economics is attractive to them if it can help improve the allocation of health resources, increase their efficiency, identify more cost-effective technologies and reduce waste (Kleczkowski 1980).

These various strands can be brought together to indicate why health economics is likely to be of increasing significance in the developing world:

(1) an economic climate where resources are extremely scarce and decisions on priorities are crucial but difficult;
(2) a growing appreciation among health professionals and policy-makers that health economics and economists can help them formulate policies and make decisions;
(3) the increasing maturity of the sub-discipline of health economics; and
(4) the growth of interest among economists and others in applying their economic skills to health issues.

None the less, there is often a lack of knowledge among politicians, government officials, health administrators, and health professionals on what health economics is, and what it can and cannot do. Most applied economists have had the experience of being taken as glorified cost accountants, cost–benefit calculators, hatchet-men, or rubber-stampers of projects. As a group, economists may be seen as *aficionados* of the market place, or as revolutionaries seeking to establish the rule of economics. A clear exposition of the health economist's approach and contribution to the health sector is required: that, in essence, is the aim of this book.

The scope of the book

All the contributors have been selected for their direct knowledge and recent experience of working in developing countries, and for their ability to illuminate the ways in which economic concepts and techniques can be, and are being, applied to health and health services. Their aim is to indicate both the present scope of applied economic analysis and the potential of economics in planning and analysing the health sector.

While the contributors have all worked, or are working, in developing countries, some for a considerable number of years, it is none the less the case that all have British or American origins. Ideally, this would be otherwise; in large part it reflects the scarcity of local health economists in developing countries and the relative advantage those economists based in developed countries enjoy in access to source material and to the latest theoretical developments in health economics. If increasing numbers of economists in the developing world are attracted into health economics, future publications will be able to reflect this growth in their choice of authors.

Turning to the content of the book, each chapter represents an attempt to review the 'state of the art' in a particular area, to consider theoretical developments, research findings, and practical applications. The book, as a whole, cannot claim to be comprehensive for at least three reasons. First, more work has been carried out on some issues than on others, a fact which a book reviewing the state of a discipline must reflect. Secondly, the scope of health economics is so broad, especially when defined to include topics on the boundaries of the health sector and linking with other sub-disciplines (such as agricultural economics, development economics), that it cannot be conveniently contained within the covers of a single volume. Thirdly, some health economics work is published and distributed world-wide (for instance WHO and World Bank publications). While these publications are cited throughout the book, the primary intention in this book was to bring together as much as possible of the less accessible and often unpublished literature of health economics.

Before outlining the scope of this book, therefore, it is useful to summarize what is not covered. Of the topics on the boundaries of health economics, the main exclusion is the international context of health: that is the involvement in developing countries of international agencies and their influence; the significance and nature of health aid; and the role of multinational companies supplying the health sector, especially pharmaceutical companies and companies selling medical technologies. Within the health sector, the book emphasizes the broader aspects of health, and thus excludes any detailed studies of, for instance, demand functions, hospital cost functions, or health service supplies systems. Such topics are, however, analysed in theoretical terms in several of the chapters.

The overall scope and content of the book can now be laid out. This first chapter has provided an introduction to the subject of health in developing countries, in order to define its boundaries, analyse some of its concerns and to set out for the reader a brief exposition of the sub-discipline of health economics. Aspects of the historical development of health economics have been described, both to indicate the relevance of health economics to countries now in the process of development and to note some of the differences between the body of literature that has grown up on health economics issues in developed countries, and that which has been written for developing countries.

The first major issue which needs to be considered is the process of economic development itself, and the second chapter (by George Cumper) introduces a broad view of health economics by looking at the connections between economic development, health services and health. A concern common to all developing countries is their wish to accelerate their rate of economic growth and to improve the standard of living of their populations. What impact does this process, conventionally known as economic development, have on health status; which effects are favourable and which unfavourable? Moreover if, as is argued in the chapter, health constitutes an important component of increased social welfare, how can health be improved most efficiently? Responding to such a question requires an examination of the influences on, and determinants of,

the state of health of a population, including assessment of the relative importance of factors such as increased income, urbanization, nutrition, and the
provision of education, water, sanitation, and health services themselves. A prime
objective of such an investigation is to identify what scope exists for improving
health through the provision of health care independently of a country's achievement of general economic development.

This chapter can therefore assist the health planner to identify which interventions are needed to improve health, and which are likely to have the greatest
impact. A basic requirement for further work, however, is information on the
financing and expenditure of the health sector, and this issue is addressed in
Chapter 3 by Adrian Griffiths and Michael Mills. Such information, indeed, is
vital for any planning or analysis of the health sector, and clearly falls within
the area of interest and competence of health economics. Economists have been
interested in health sector financing for some time, but only recently has progress
been made in developing methodologies that can easily be used by planners and
researchers in developing countries. A substantial part of Chapter 3, therefore,
is devoted to showing how health sector financing and expenditure surveys can
be undertaken quickly and at low cost.

Chapter 3 reveals that there are numerous means of financing the health
sector. Chapter 4 is written by Anne Mills who selects one of these means,
namely health insurance, for close examination. Health insurance represents one
of the major ways in which governments, groups or individuals have sought to
cover the cost of health care; in many developing countries, a significant proportion of the resources of the health sector is derived from insurance payments,
and a few countries have been experimenting with mechanisms appropriate for
rural and relatively unindustrialized areas. The chapter surveys health insurance
systems from an economist's point of view, looking at their impact on the demand
and supply of health services, and on their efficiency and equity. A number of
criteria are presented which can be used to analyse health insurance schemes
and to indicate which particular mechanisms and features can best minimise
their adverse effects.

Health improvement strategies that can meet the needs of the large sections
of populations at present without easy access to health services also need to be
considered. Chapter 5 by Kenneth Lee examines the economic implications of
alternative approaches to improving health, and particularly the philosophy and
content of primary health care. For an economist, the most important economic
variable is 'cost', since it determines what can be done, what is deferred and
what is foregone. It influences the ways in which primary health care can be
financed, its technology and its pattern of activity. Chapter 5 thus looks at a
number of key economic issues that arise in securing resources for, and meeting
the costs of, primary health care. It also provides a list of questions to help
policy-makers and planners evaluate their primary care policies and services.

The study of primary health care raises many issues about manpower training,
mix, and cost. In Chapter 6, these issues are considered in more detail by

Geoffrey Ferster and Robert Tilden. Expenditure on manpower is usually the largest single category of health expenditure in any country. Moreover, a nation's human resources are essential inputs to the development process. Policies on manpower development are thus crucial, and a key to the improvement of health status is the education, training, and motivation of a range of health workers, from health professionals to community volunteers. Chapter 6 therefore examines what manpower policy approaches might be most effective and efficient in tackling the health manpower problems faced by developing countries. It considers questions such as the manpower policy-making and planning process, the scope for decentralization of manpower planning, the use of community workers, the operation of the labour market, determinants of the demand for and supply of health workers, and finally, the influences affecting the motivations of health workers.

All chapters so far have considered, amongst other things, the relative merits of different options, whether they be for improving health, financing health services, or training health manpower. The formal evaluation or appraisal of such options forms the subject of Chapter 7, written by Nicholas Prescott and Jeremy Warford. Rather than focusing on any one specific health activity, the authors describe and explain economic techniques of appraisal that can be applied to any public investment decision in the health sector. Such techniques, designed to maximise the achievement of social objectives and increase the efficiency of public expenditure, have in the past been widely used outside the health sector but very little within it. By explaining the techniques of cost-benefit and cost–effectiveness analysis of health programmes and showing how these have been applied, the authors demonstrate that there is considerable scope for their use in the future.

Chapter 8 (by Andrew Creese) also considers economic evaluation, by showing how the approach has been applied to a particular activity, namely immunization. Immunization has many advocates: it represents a preventive measure that is directed at major sources of morbidity and mortality and that can be highly effective. However, the relative priority to be given to immunization in comparison to other life-saving investments, and what strategies might deliver effective immunizations at least cost, are not only relatively unexplored topics, but also issues of central concern to health economists. The advantage of selecting immunization for special attention is that its characteristics make it possible to apply economic evaluation more rigorously than is at present possible in some other areas of primary health care.

Most chapters in this book concentrate either on the health sector itself or on services contained within it. In Chapter 9, Gill Westcott looks outside the sector, to an area identified in Chapter 2 as being of significance to health, namely nutrition. Problems relating to nutrition underlie much of the pattern of childhood morbidity and mortality in developing countries. It is thus an area that health planners, policy-makers, and economists must be aware of and understand. Nutrition planning also provides the opportunity to draw upon some of the concepts and techniques described in previous chapters, and to add some other aspect of economics, such as the determination of food prices, consumption patterns, and production. In addition, the chapter considers the ways in which nutritional objectives can be incorporated into both health and general development planning.

This subject leads logically to Chapter 10, by Mark Wheeler, on the relationship between health sector planning and development planning. Development economics has formulated a number of models to optimize the allocation of resources within an economy; these are often used as the basis for development planning. Such models, however, are rarely suited to the health sector; they typically leave it to optimize its own objectives within resource constraints laid down by central planners. Moreover, while health sector planning has taken a variety of forms, few of them are well placed to take account of the links between health and economic development. The chapter thus picks up the theme, introduced in Chapter 2, of how these links can be incorporated in the health planning process.

The final chapter, by Kenneth Lee and Anne Mills, provides a critical review of the role of economists and economics in the formulation and implementation of health policies. Its intention is both to pull together the various strands of the book, and to review the scope of health economics. It includes a glossary of economic concepts and also notes some of the conceptual and methodological problems economists face in applying these ideas to the health sector. Economists are often accused (sometimes justifiably) of having a naïve view of organizational and political realities, and of expecting individuals and organizations to obey the laws of economic rationality. Lee and Mills also discuss, therefore, the political and institutional constraints to the acceptance of economic analysis in the health sector, and the processes by which economic analysis can most effectively be incorporated into policy-making and planning in developing countries.

Conclusion

A number of common themes run through the various chapters of this book. One is the provision of an analytical framework to help ensure that a country's scarce resources, and those resources available to the health sector, are allocated in such a way as to maximize their contribution to national objectives and social welfare. Another theme is that the concerns of health economics should be tailored to the particular needs and circumstances of developing countries; for instance by exploring the economic notions of efficiency, effectiveness, and equity, and the ways in which economics can help to analyse these concepts and determine the extent to which they are being achieved in practice. All the chapters aim also to demonstrate the assistance economics and economists can provide in adapting health strategies to the circumstances of particular countries.

Finally, each chapter attempts to translate the professional language of economics into a form which allows the lay reader to comprehend policy and planning issues from an economic perspective. In consequence, the tone of the book is that of applied economics, and the chapters attempt to ask and answer questions of real relevance to health policy-makers, planners, and professionals throughout the developing world.

REFERENCES

Abel-Smith, B. (1976). *Value for money in health services*. Heinemann, London.
— and Leiserson, A. (1978). Poverty, development and health policy. *Publ. Hlth Pap. WHO* **69**.
Brandt Commission (1980). *North–South: a programme for survival*. Pan Books, London.
Culyer, A. J. (1981). Health, economics and health economics. In *Health, economics and health economics* (ed. J. van der Gaag and M. Perlman). North-Holland, Amsterdam.
— Wiseman, J., and Walker, A. (1977). *An annotated bibliography of health economics*. Martin Robertson, Oxford.
Cumper, G. (1982). Social and organisational constraints on health development. *J. trop. Med. Hyg.* **85**, 47–55.
Djukanovic, V. and Mach, E. P. (ed.) (1975). *Alternative approaches to meeting basic health needs in developing countries*. World Health Organization, Geneva.
Duke, B. O. L. (1981). The six diseases of WHO: Lymphatic and other filariases. *Br. med. J.* **283**, 1036–7.
Fein, R. (1980). Social and economic attitudes shaping American health policy. *Milbank meml Fund Q. Bull.* (Health and Society) **58**, 349–85.
Fox, D. M. (1979). From reform to relativism: A history of economists and health care. *Milbank meml Fund Q. Bull.* **57**, 297–336.
Giles, B. D. (1979). Economists in government: The case of Malawi. *J. Develop. Stud.* **15**, 216–32.
Gilles, H. M. (1981). The six diseases of WHO: Malaria. *Br. med. J.* **283**, 1382–5.
Gish, O. (1975). *Planning the health sector: The Tanzanian experience*. Croom Helm, London.
Griffiths, A. and Bankowski, Z. (ed.) (1980). *Economics and health policy*, The Council for International Organizations of Medical Sciences (CIOMS) and Sandoz Institute, Geneva.
Griffiths, D. A. T., Rigoni, R., Tacier, P., and Prescott, N. M. (1980). *An annotated bibliography of health economics: Western European sources*. Published for Sandoz Institute for Health and Socio-Economic Studies, Geneva, by Martin Robertson, Oxford.
Gwatkin, D. R., Wilcox, J. R., and Wray, J. D. (1980). The policy implications of field experiments in primary health and nutrition care. *Social sci. med.* **14C**, 121–8.
Klarman, H. E. (1979). Health economics and health economics research. *Milbank mem. Fund Q. Bull.* **57**, 371–9.
Kleczkowski, B. M. (1980). Technological imperatives and economic efficiency in health care. In *Economics and health policy* (ed. A. Griffiths and Z. Bankowski). The Council for International Organizations of Medical Sciences (CIOMS) and Sandoz Institute, Geneva.
Knodel, J. and Chamratrithirong, A. (1977). Infant and child mortality in Thailand. (Mimeo.)
Lee, K. and Mills, A. J. (1979*a*). The contribution of economics to health service planning. *Hlth Soc. Service J.* (Centre 8 papers) **4627**, C35–40.

— — (1979*b*). The role of economists and economics in health service planning: A general overview. In *Economics and health planning* (ed. K. Lee). Croom Helm, London.

Livingstone, I. (1981). The development of development economics. *ODI Rev.* 2, 1–19.

Mills, A. J. (1975). Results of a study of expenditure on health care in Malawi. (Mimeo.) Ministry of Health, Malawi.

NSO (National Statistical Office) (1977). Survey of population change. (Mimeo.) National Statistical Office, Thailand.

Prescott, N. M. (1979). The economics of malaria, filariasis and human trypano-somiasis. Document TDR/SER(SC-1)/80.4. World Health Organization, Geneva.

Rosenthal, G. (1979). Of economists and economics, *ceteris paribus*. *Milbank meml. Fund Q. Bull.* 57, 291–6.

Russell, P. F. and Menon, M. K. (1942). A malario–economic survey in rural South India. *Indian Med. Gaz.* 77, 167–80.

Samuelson, P. A. (1976). *Economics*, 10th edn. McGraw-Hill, New York.

Seers, D. (1969). *The meaning of development*. Eleventh World Conference of the Society for International Development, New Delhi.

Sinton, J. A. (1935). What malaria costs India, nationally, socially, economically. *Rec. Malar. Surv. India* 5, 223–64, 413–89.

— (1936). What malaria costs India, nationally, socially, economically. *Rec. Malar. Surv. India* 6, 96–169.

Sorkin, A. (1976). *Health economics in developing countries*, Lexington Books, D. C. Heath & Co., Lexington, Mass.

Streeten, P. (1979). How poor are the poor countries and why? *The frontiers of development studies*, Chapter 3. Macmillan, London.

Todaro, M. P. (1977). *Economic development in the Third World*. Longman, London.

Van Dine, D. L. (1916). The relation of malaria to crop production. *Scient. Mon., NY*. November 431–9.

Webbe, G. (1981). The six diseases of WHO: Schistosomiasis. *Br. med. J.* 283, 1104–6.

Williams, A. (1980). Economics and health care. *Int. J. Epidemiol.* 9, 296–8.

World Bank (1980*a*) *World development report 1980*. World Bank, Washington DC.

— (1980*b*). *Health: sector policy paper*. World Bank, Washington DC.

— (1981*a*). *World development report 1981*. Oxford University Press, New York.

— (1981*b*). *Accelerated development in sub-Saharan Africa: an agenda for action*. World Bank, Washington DC.

WHO (World Health Organization) (1975). Health economics. *Publ. Hlth Pap. WHO*, No. 64.

— (1978). The financing of health services. *Tech. Rep. Ser. Wld Hlth Org.* 625.

— (1981). The world's main health problems. *World Health Forum* 2, 264–80.

2

Economic development, health services, and health

George Cumper

Introduction

It would be widely agreed that there is likely to be an association between a country's place on the ladder of development and its health status. To be useful for planning purposes, this association needs to be defined more precisely. This chapter concentrates on two aspects of the association: the ways in which economic development promotes (or, sometimes, impairs) the health status of the population undergoing development; and the scope for health improvement through the provision of health care independently of a country's achievement of general economic development. The following sections deal with the concept of economic development; the association of development with changing levels of health; hypotheses about the relationships underlying this association; ways of testing these hypotheses; the results of some important studies in this field; and a statement of the conclusions which can be drawn from these and other studies. Many of the points introduced in this chapter are discussed more fully in later chapters.

The meaning of development

It is now about 40 years since the word 'development' came into common use as a label for certain recognizable and important processes of economic and social change. 'Development', in this sense, has proved easier to recognize than to define; its meaning has shifted from decade to decade, and at a given time has tended to be different for different groups—academics, planners, administrators —and different individuals. The common ground has been a concern with establishing, theoretically and practically, the conditions for a continuing increase in the welfare of human populations. But there have been significant changes in the consensus about which conditions were necessary, sufficient, or both, and which aspects of welfare deserved most attention. These changes help to explain the increasing role of health in the last decade in the theory and practice of development.

In the 1940s and 1950s, the central problem of development was seen as one of increasing material production (and hence a matter for the economist, agronomist, and engineer). This point of view did not, as is sometimes alleged, imply hardness of heart, wilful blindness, or a political commitment to market economics. The emphasis on material production was common to both capitalist and socialist theories of growth, as can be seen from the nature of the early Russian assistance to independent India. The leading development economists were clear that increased material production was a necessary, but not a sufficient, condition for greater welfare. Such production made available to the government of a country resources uncommitted to consumption, of which a portion could be used for social purposes; guidance on what these should be could be found in the economics of welfare and its applications in the field of public finance. But the resources available for social purposes were limited in two ways. Since they represented a subtraction from the surplus available for investment, they reduced the rate of growth of material production in the future; hence fixing too high a level of social expenditure too early in the development process would be self-defeating. Further, in the case of a market economy there would be theoretical limits on social measures directed toward achieving a more equal distribution of income, for the excess of the incomes of the rich over their consumption needs was expected to be the main source of finance for investment.

In practice, the formulation of development plans, and still more their implementation, were less Spartan than the theory would lead one to believe. But it was generally true that emphasis was placed on 'economic' expenditures, designed to increase the stock of physical capital which was seen as the main instrument of growth. In these circumstances, health received little of planners' funds or attention, and remained something of a backwater. Much more of both money and effort was devoted to a frontal attack on what was seen as the more urgent problem of population control.

The grand simplicities of early development theory began to disintegrate in the 1960s. This was not necessarily because it had failed in its own terms: most poor countries were achieving a rate of growth of incomes which stayed ahead of the rate of population increase, even though the latter fell less rapidly than had been hoped. But it began to be appreciated that for many countries the existing development strategies would take many years to produce significant effects on welfare—a prospect which imperial powers could face more stoically than the governments of newly independent countries. A series of new elements were introduced into development theory, some of which favoured a greater role for health.

One such element was the introduction into development theory of a more realistic view of the production function, and particularly the acceptance of the concept of 'human capital'. Early development theory, stripped down to essentials, saw output as a function of the quantity of three factors—land, labour, and capital— of which the first could be ignored in analyses of the crucial industrial sector. Labour was interpreted, in terms which would have been familiar to Ricardo and Marx, as a pool of undifferentiated labour power which was assumed to be in unlimited supply; hence the primacy of capital— again given a simple physical interpretation—as a determinant of growth. In practice, the quality of labour proved to be important even on a mechanistic view of production, and some aspects of quality could be plausibly connected with the health of the present and future work force. The connection proved hard to demonstrate specifically, but this did not prevent its acceptance in general terms.

Another element was the increased attention given to measures of social welfare. Early development theory got by without much use of data on national incomes—necessarily, since such data were only just becoming familiar in developed countries and in most developing countries were simply unavailable. In the 1950s and 1960s the number of countries with national accounting systems increased greatly, but almost immediately the resulting estimates of national income and product came under more and more critical scrutiny. Their limitations as measures of welfare directed attention to the possibility of supplementing them with indicators for social factors such as employment, education, and health.

Finally, one of the harshest features of early development theory was the constraints it placed on any measures to equalize the distribution of incomes. These constraints were morally repugnant and politically inconvenient; experience suggested that they were also in part unnecessary, since high incomes were not always a reliable source of finance for productive investment. Hence a legitimate place was found, even in market economics, for social mechanisms to equalize the welfare gains from development, of which a wider distribution of health benefits could be one.

Thus, in the 1960s, there was increasing scepticism about investment in physical capital, increasing attention to direct measures of social welfare, and increasing concern about the effect of development measures on equity. These are three of the reasons why in the mid-1970s the stage was set for versions of the development drama in which health would play a more prominent role; other reasons could be cited, including the honourable ambitions of health professionals at the national and international levels to make their distinctive contribution to development. What is relevant to the present chapter is that the script for this drama was, and is, far from clear. What form of development theory and practice will contribute most efficiently to improving the health of the populations of developing countries? An answer to this question must rest, first, on some analysis of the determinants of health, and secondly on an assessment of these determinants in terms of their susceptibility to control through planning and purposeful change.

To make such an enquiry feasible it is necessary to define health in a way which separates it from other aspects of welfare. In this chapter health is taken to be that part of human welfare which depends on the normal functioning of the body. It would be generally accepted that the health of a population, so defined, is influenced by a wide range of economic and social variables, including many which change markedly in the course of development. But one can make a broad distinction between variables such as the level of health services, where the connection with health is intentional and direct; other variables where the connection is well established though not a matter of primary intention, such as the level of literacy; and variables whose effect on health levels is diffuse and uncertain, though possibly important, such as patterns of housing. Where, on this continuum, the emphasis is placed will affect not only the choice of strategy for development in the health field, but also which national and international agencies are to be responsible for its implementation and what their roles should be. Stress on the first type of variable will strengthen the position of agencies controlled by health professionals (ministries of health on the national scale, and the World Health Organization at the international level). Stress on the second and third types will increase the responsibility of agencies with a broader remit such as national planning bodies. This is an additional reason for taking seriously the analysis of the determinants of health.

Development and changing levels of health

In trying to identify those aspects of development which can be manipulated so as to improve the health situation in developing countries, the most promising starting point is the experience of the countries which have been classed as 'developing' in the period since about 1940. History can show many earlier examples of economic development, each no doubt with its correlates in terms of changing levels of health; but the further one moves into the past, the weaker the data becomes and the more alien the economic, social, and technical context. The countries now classed as 'developed' enter the picture as one end of the income continuum, but their current health experience has to be treated with caution as a guide to what the developing countries can expect. This section outlines the general relationships between economic development, health services, and health as it appears from the recent historical record. Later sections consider the techniques available for more intensive analysis of this relationship, particularly those using economic models, and the results of some applications of these techniques.

Given a body of historical data on a population (in this case, a set of countries) passing through the same set of processes, there is in principle a choice between interpreting the data synchronically or diachronically—that is, in terms of differences between countries at one point in time, or between the situation of a single country at successive times. The synchronic approach is used more often in this section, because the necessary data are more abundant. This requires that one asks first how far the synchronic and diachronic approaches are likely to agree: are the processes involved in economic and health development stable, or has their structure shifted over the period of concern?

It is useful to start by taking as an indicator of development the crude but serviceable measure of per capita national income. On this measure, most countries of the world in the post-war period have experienced development. For any given country, the process has not been uniform over time, and some countries (often those with special problems of political stability) have fallen badly behind the rest, while others (such as the 'newly industrialized countries', e.g. Singapore, South Korea) have moved ahead. Nevertheless, the rate of real income growth (in terms, for example, of percentage increase in GNP per annum) has been within a fairly narrow range for most countries at most periods, leaving the average income level world-wide in the 1970s substantially higher than in, say, 1950, and the international distribution of incomes not greatly changed. Have these differences in income level, over time or between countries, been associated with predictable differences in economic structure?

In broad terms the answer is clearly 'yes'. This is reassuring since any other answer would cast doubt on the validity of the whole concept of economic development. Historically or comparatively, economies which have higher income levels also tend to be more capital-intensive, to depend on secondary industry rather than agriculture or person-to-person services, to devote less of their consumption activities to food and less of their food expenditure to basic carbohydrates—to name only some obvious trends. National paths to economic development do differ according to physical endowment and changes in the international context. Furthermore, the technological content of a particular category of production or consumption is not the same in 1980 as it was in 1950. But for the present purposes, the common features are more important than the differences.

This remains true if the picture is broadened to incorporate differences in social structure. To take first some of the more easily measurable characteristics, richer countries tend to be more urbanized and to have higher literacy rates than poor ones. Generalizations about cultural factors are harder to establish, but it is arguable that richer countries are more individualistic and, in some sense, rationalistic than poorer ones. Again, the association of higher incomes with certain social and cultural features is not a mechanistic one, and development cannot simply be identified with a single process of 'modernization'. Further, wherever a social variable has a technological content (e.g. education), that content cannot be taken to be the same now as in 1950. But there is a definable core of social change associated with economic development whether looked at diachronically or synchronically.

Can the same be said of the association between development and health? There is certainly a tendency for differences in income between countries, or over time, to correspond to differences in the indicators of health status and also of the availability of health services. Using standard indicators such as Infant Mortality Rate (IMR) or Life Expectancy at Birth (LEB), about two-thirds of the international variance in health status can be connected with income differences (see, for example, Grosse 1980; Preston 1975). The poorest countries at present show IMRs of about 200 per thousand live births and LEBs of about 40 years, against 10 per thousand and 75 years in the richest countries. Historical trends are harder to demonstrate but appear to follow the same general pattern. On the other hand, there are sufficient exceptions to show that the link between income and health status is not a deterministic one. There are 'poor' countries with relatively high health status (e.g. Sri Lanka) and 'rich' countries with unfavourable health indicators (e.g. Saudi Arabia). Moreover, as Preston (1975) has argued, any function connecting national income and health levels has to be thought of as shifting over time, presumably as a result of improvements in the information embodied in medical science, technology, and public education.

There is also evidence to show that development brings changes not only in the level of mortality, but in its structure (and presumably also in that of morbidity). The high mortality in poor countries reflects the high prevalence of communicable diseases (particularly diarrhoeal and respiratory diseases) and the interaction of these with malnutrition, especially among children; in richer countries, mortality from these causes is much reduced, leaving a hard core of deaths from congenital, chronic, and degenerative conditions and from external causes. These trends can be traced from both historical and comparative data.

The provision of health care services is clearly greater and access to them more equitable in richer countries than in poor ones. Using comparative data, one can show that health care expenditure forms an increasing proportion of consumption expenditure as one moves from poor to richer countries (about 3 per cent of Final Consumption Expenditure in the poorest and 10 per cent in the richest countries). Part of the increase represents the higher cost of health personnel in developed countries, but the increase in real per capita inputs is still very great, as can be shown from comparative data on the numbers of hospital beds, physicians, and other health workers in relation to population. Such historical data as is available generally confirms these trends. But it is evident that there have been considerable technological shifts over the period since the 1940s, both in curative (e.g. antibiotics) and preventive (e.g. DDT) medicine.

Thus, whether the analysis is based on comparative or historical data, the broad picture is one in which the indicators of economic, social, and health development tend to move together. If a quietist attitude is taken to health development, regarding it as secondary to economic development, this picture is a consoling one; it suggests that substantial improvements in global levels of health will follow as a natural result of favourable economic changes. During the 1960s and 1970s, however, a more activist approach gained ground which called for specific action to maximize the welfare effects of development, to bring about improvements in welfare even though the process of income growth may falter. In the health field, this approach calls for a much closer examination of the causes of improvements in health. The parallel movements in the economic, social, and health indicators are, from this point of view, an impediment to analysis, since they mean that so many of the relevant variables are closely correlated in the historical and comparative data. More rigorous techniques of analysis than simple correlation are needed (some of which are explored in the following sections) and more attention devoted to the cases which do not fit the pattern of simultaneous economic, social, and health development.

To break away from the Panglossian view that health inevitably improves with economic development, one must look first at the conspicuous exceptions which are already established in the literature. Some of these concern the unfavourable effects on health of particular development projects (e.g. the spread of schistosomiasis as an unintended by-product of irrigation). Others involve the broader effects of development at the physical level (e.g. the effect of the use of DDT in agriculture on insecticide-resistance in mosquitoes). Others relate to the broad social effects of development (e.g. changes in diet resulting from a shift from subsistence to cash farming). Indeed, the effect of changes in diet on health has been a fertile field for theories whose status ranges from the generally accepted (the effect of saturated fats on some types of heart disease) to the speculative (the effect of lack of fibre in the diet in promoting some types of cancer). Whatever the status of particular examples, there is enough evidence to establish that unfavourable effects of development on health occur, and that in many cases they can be avoided by better planning.

Of equal interest are the cases where the health status of a developing country is substantially better or worse than would be expected on the basis of its level of economic development. These cases are most valuable in suggesting those aspects of the connection between health and development which need to be investigated by more rigorous methods. For example, a number of oil-exporting countries have high per capita national incomes and fairly high levels of conventional health service inputs together with unfavourable indicators of levels of health. Is this because incomes are very unequally distributed, because they have not yet built up an adequate infrastructure of general social services and public information about health matters, or because their populations are still suffering from the unfavourable social and environmental conditions they experienced in the past? Regression analyses using international data (Cumper, in press) suggest that island nations have a much higher level of health than their incomes would lead one to expect; is this a consequence of insularity, or to be explained case by case in terms of other factors? Is the surprisingly favourable health situation of Sri Lanka to be explained in terms of the scale of its health services, the strength of its social infrastructure, particularly education and food subsidies, or some other factor(s)? Questions like these cannot be answered by inspection or intuition. They call, first, for a systematic statement of the likely causal relationships between health and other factors; and secondly, for the application of more rigorous techniques to test the hypotheses such a statement generates. These are the subjects of the next two sections.

Hypotheses about the links between development and health

If one defines health in terms of the functioning or malfunctioning of certain physiological processes, the influence of development on health can be seen in two stages; how development affects these processes in themselves, and how it affects their translation into welfare terms. The physiological processes involved are very diverse, but they can be classed for the present purpose into broad groups with common characteristics:

— growth and development, from conception to physical maturity;
— malfunctioning connected with an external pathogen (mainly the communicable diseases, including respiratory conditions);
— the effects of trauma (accidents and violence);
— processes connected with maternity (pregnancy, childbirth, lactation); and,
— degenerative processes not primarily due to any of the above.

The first question is how are these processes affected at the physical level by the basic features of economic development? The ways in which the external environment can impinge on the functioning of the human body are rather limited; they involve the intake of food and water, invasion by pathogens, or what may loosely be called stress—exposure to values of variables such as temperature, humidity, and noise which fall outside tolerable limits. Two of the groups of processes set out above—degenerative processes and trauma—are not very sensitive to these external factors over the range of variation found in developing countries, and play little part in determining differences in health status from one country to another. Therefore, one can concentrate for the moment on the other three groups.

How will these be affected by economic development? If only an increase in average income is considered, without regard to the structure of development, there is clearly a strong possibility that the external factors will become more favourable to health. Higher incomes permit more, and more varied, food, more water, and a reduction of stress through better clothing and housing, and experience shows that they will be spent in just those ways. There are two caveats to this conclusion. One is that the distribution of individual incomes must not become more unequal as the average increases. The evidence on the relationship between development and income distribution is conflicting, and it may be that there is no deterministic connection at all. The other caution is that a sufficient proportion of any increase in incomes must be available for collective action to control environmental factors which cannot be dealt with at the individual level—for example, mosquito control.

If the changes in economic structure which usually go with development are brought into the picture—for example, the shift from agriculture to industry—there is little reason to believe that on balance they are either favourable or unfavourable to health. There may be some reduction in the incidence of communicable diseases connected with agriculture—for example schistosomiasis—but these have to be weighed against possible increases in stress and other industrial health problems.

There are some social changes which accompany economic development so regularly that any analysis must take into account their effect on health. Three of them are considered here—urbanization, the substitution of cash for subsistence production, and the spread of formal education. They present something of a paradox. All can be thought of as favouring health—urbanization, for instance, because it makes more economic the provision of certain centralized services; monetization, because it facilitates cash payments for individual or collective health care; education, as a basis for appropriate health action by the public. But the first two, at least, could be cited in the opposite sense. Urbanization may lower the quality of the environment, for instance, by bringing individuals and households closer together, and so increasing the level of transmission of certain communicable diseases; the shift away from subsistence production can lead to an impoverished diet. This introduces a new theme which is important for the argument of the rest of the chapter; that many aspects of development cannot be classified as being favourable or unfavourable *per se* to health, but should rather be seen as having a wide range of possible effects, with the ultimate outcome depending on positive action if development is to promote health. This positive action has often to be collective in nature. There is a further lesson to be drawn; a particular aspect of development does not affect all types of health process in the same direction, and its net effect on indicators such as mortality or morbidity will reflect both favourable and unfavourable effects.

At the same time, there are some interactions which are usually presumed to be almost wholly unfavourable to health. One can make a plausible connection between the stresses of development and the fact that with higher incomes a constant or increasing proportion of expenditure is on anodynes of various kinds—alcohol, tobacco, coca, ganja, qat, etc.—whose net effect on health is almost certainly negative. This is a particularly interesting area because the causal relationships are so difficult to define: should the negative health effects be attributed to the availability of the consumer good in question, or to higher incomes, or to the development process *per se*?

Thus, even in terms of the physiological effects of the changing environment produced by development, account has to be taken of a complex network of relationships. Unfortunately, there are further considerations which raise the complexity to an even higher power. One is that the welfare implications of a given physiological state may themselves be changed by development processes. Pregnancy and childbirth, for example, have very different welfare implications according to the degree of social support the mother can expect, and this may be much less in an urbanized setting than in an integrated rural community. Disabilities only take on meaning in relation to the tasks to be performed, and these will vary between different development contexts. Yet, it may well be possible by purposeful action—provision of maternal and child health services, or of prostheses, for example—to compensate for any welfare loss from developmental changes, and still attain a higher level of welfare.

The final level of sophistication comes when account is taken of the fact that all the processes referred to above are locked into economic, social, and demographic systems which have their own conditions of equilibrium and growth, at all levels from the household to the nation and the international community. Thus, at the level of the household budget, health care expenditure competes with food expenditure, producing indirect effects which may be important; or at the national level, reductions in mortality may raise the rate of population increase, depress average incomes, and exert pressure on the budget for social services.

In the above argument it has been implicitly assumed that no genetic factors need to be taken into account. It would be true to say that genetic factors do influence health, but there is little evidence that they interact with development, except in two fields. One is the existence of a hereditary component in certain diseases which are concentrated in populations in countries at low levels of economic development (e.g. sickle cell anaemia). So far, such diseases do not appear to be quantitatively important in the global health picture. A second topic, broader but more difficult to investigate, is the place of genetic factors in human growth and development. The populations of poor countries are generally smaller and lighter, age for age, than those of richer ones. Much of the difference is clearly associated with levels of nutrition, particularly in childhood, since there is evidence that differences in stature between groups can be reduced or eliminated by better nutrition and general health care. But the possibility cannot be entirely excluded that genetic factors may interact with nutrition in determining the mechanical and intellectual efficiency of populations.

In summary, development affects health in a complex way. Its overall effect is to make more resources available to deal with health problems. At the same time, particular aspects of development affect particular physiological and welfare components of health and may be favourable and unfavourable. Commonly, development creates a range of possibilities out of which the most favourable can be selected by purposeful action. This action may or may not be included in the provision of health services as usually defined, but will usually include some minimum component of collective action.

Testing the hypotheses: available techniques

Given the complexity of the relationships between development, health services, and health status, it is evident that any testable hypothesis must be concerned with some subset of these relationships. Different investigators have concentrated on different subsets, depending on the kind of problem which has aroused their interest, their professional field, and the availability of data. (The following section gives some examples of investigations which involve economics and related disciplines.) It should be borne in mind that the investigation of most problems in this field depends, at some remove, on the results of work in the natural sciences. Much of this uses classical experimental techniques; that is, the testing of hypotheses through the controlled manipulation of an experimental situation. These techniques can rarely be applied to the investigation of the economic and social aspects of the health system. The studies discussed below therefore depend on the application of observational rather than experimental techniques to the health and development fields.

The non-availability of data is one of the main limitations at present on the use of such observational techniques. Some investigations rely on existing standard series developed for administrative and statistical purposes; the quality of these, and particularly their international comparability, is greater in the economic and demographic fields than in health. Other investigations include the generation of the specific data required and its analysis within a single project. However, an important contribution to the testing of hypotheses about health and development can be made through the improvement of the quality of the required statistics (e.g. WHO's work on health statistics) or through the collection and publication of data which experience has shown to be of general utility to scientists and the public, even though such data are not tied to a specific, current project (e.g. the World Fertility Surveys). Unfortunately, large scale prospective studies and the building of data banks are usually national rather than international in scope and are rare in developing countries. In this context, an important contribution to the development of basic international data may come from the promotion by WHO of studies of national health expenditure and the application of the results to health planning (see, for example, Abel-Smith 1967; Abel-Smith and Leiserson 1978).

Observational studies relevant to health and development have tended to fall into two groups: those concerned with single diseases and conditions, and those concerned with some overall indicator of health status (IMR, LEB). In each case the main concern has been to demonstrate an association between health and some external factor, whether in the economic and social setting, the health service context, or both. But the precision with which the association has been specified, and the sophistication of the techniques used to verify it, have varied greatly. Particularly in the case of single diseases and conditions, the early exploratory work has often been based on scattered statistics and reports, evaluated intuitively (e.g. the association between salt intake and hypertension, or breast-feeding and infant mortality). If the original hypothesis holds up at this level, a process of more rigorous testing begins which involves a more specific statement of the association, more systematic data collection, more rigorous statistical analysis and more co-ordination between observational and experimental investigations. In some cases the methods of medical geography have been used to generate and test hypotheses.

Macro-level studies using broad indicators of health levels and other variables have tended to make heavy use of regression techniques. Two-variable regressions using ordinary least squares have often been the starting point. But the application of simple regression techniques to complex situations is liable to yield paradoxical results (see, for example, Cochrane, St. Leger, and Moore 1978; St. Leger, Cochrane, and Moore 1978). In some cases, investigators have therefore turned to multiple regressions and more sophisticated approaches such as discriminant and path analysis. The underlying model has initially usually been one of simple linear association without detailed specification of the physical processes involved, and although models have become more complex with continuing investigation, the links with the natural sciences have so far been sketchier than in the case of epidemiological models of single disease problems.

The ultimate test of a hypothesis is its power of prediction. In investigating the relation between development and health, this power cannot be tested in its classical experimental form—the prediction of behaviour of an otherwise controlled system when a single variable is manipulated. Apart from data limitations and ethical problems, the system under scrutiny is much more complex than any model that can presently be specified, and one variable can rarely be changed in isolation from the rest. How, for example, can income be changed without changing expenditure on health care, and conversely? But there may still be value in a quasi-experimental approach under which change is induced and its results analysed with as full allowance as possible for the uncontrolled elements—as in, for example, the study of the effects on health status of improvements in health care, carried out at Narangwal, Punjab, by a group from Johns Hopkins University (see Gwatkin, Wilcox, and Wray 1980).

Some illustrative studies

This chapter does not attempt to offer a full review of the literature on the relationship between economic development and health. The field is too broad, ill-defined, and complex, and the results obtained so far too inconclusive, to make this worth while. Instead, this section reviews six studies dealing with various aspects of this relationship. They have been chosen primarily because of the importance of the topics they deal with and secondarily for the light they throw on methodological problems.

Income, health, and technical progress

The question of the stability of the relation between mortality and economic development (defined in terms of per capita income) has been addressed directly by Preston, using relatively simple statistical techniques, in a study which raises important substantive issues (Preston 1975). A logistic curve is fitted to each of two sets of national data on life expectancy and per capita income, one set for the 1930s, the other for the 1960s. The curves are steepest at low levels of per capita income, suggesting that in poor countries a given increase in incomes brings a much greater absolute improvement in life expectancy than in the richer ones; and the curve for the 1960s is parallel to, but consistently above, that for the 1930s. Hence, countries which experienced both an income increase and an increase in life expectancy between these two dates would have benefited from two effects; one linking health to income, the other leading to an improvement in health independent of the change in the country's income level. Preston estimates that on the world scale the second effect much outweighed the first. Parallel calculations using 1976 data suggest that the shift in the income–health relationship continued up to that date. What is the nature of this non-income effect?

While Preston does not attempt an exhaustive answer to this question, he produces evidence against some of the obvious ways in which economic and social factors other than changes in health services might have increased life expectancy, such as increases in literacy and better nutrition. Further, the mortality situation of socialist countries for a given income level appears worse than the average, suggesting that equality of income distribution is not an important factor. Hence it is argued that the shift in the relation of income to health is due in large part to the spread of medical knowledge and technology, whether in the form of curative or preventive medicine or greater public knowledge about health. (One example cited in this connection is the control of malaria in countries such as Guyana and Sri Lanka, referred to further below.)

Preston's argument is of particular interest for health economics because it suggests an analogy between the improvement of health technology and the spread of innovation in more conventional fields of production. It therefore opens up the possibility of applying models of technical progress, already developed for agriculture and industry, to the provision of health care. It also raises the question whether the processes involved should be seen entirely in terms of current flows of inputs and outputs (as is usual), or partly in terms of the building up of stocks—stocks of information, of material goods, and of the former incorporated in the latter or in people. A stock approach, particularly in relation to public information, would help to explain some extreme cases of disproportion between mortality and health inputs—for example, the high mortality experience of some rich oil-exporting countries. It would also have the important implication that improvements in health may not be symmetrically reversible. The fact that for some decades increases in incomes and in the inputs of various social services have gone along on the average with improvements in health, would not necessarily mean that these improvements would cease if incomes and social inputs ceased to grow—a point of obvious topical importance in the present depressed state of the world economy.

Income, social inputs, and health: a multiple regression approach

The adoption by the international agencies in the late 1970s of 'health for all by the year 2000' as a policy for immediate implementation, and its endorsement by national governments (not all of which were tongue in cheek), carried with it two assumptions important to the present chapter. One was that health improvements in developing countries could be brought about by social policy independently of general increases in incomes, through means such as better health services, education, nutrition, water supply, and sanitation. The other was that such improvements could be carried out within the resource constraints of the poor countries, through increased external assistance, transfers of resources from other uses, or greater efficiency in resource use. The writer became involved in an investigation of these assumptions, first while on the staff of WHO and later independently. The results of the first stage of the investigation were presented to a WHO seminar on the costs and financing of primary health care (Cumper 1980) and prompted further work, the results of which are reported below.

It is easy to establish that a wide range of social inputs—health services, education, nutrition, water supply, and sanitation—show strong simple correlations with per capita income, with indicators of health status and with each other. This can be demonstrated at the international level, in some cases for subnational groupings, and in terms of plausible mechanisms affecting the individual. Once a body of comparative international data had been established, the obvious next step was to use multiple regression techniques to assess the association of each category of social input with health status, with other factors (including per capita income) held constant. The infant mortality rate was used as the best indicator of national health status. The available data on nutrition were judged unsatisfactory, and nutrition was therefore not treated as a separate variable, its effects presumably being absorbed into those of income (along with those of other variables which could in principle have been treated as social inputs, such as housing). Income distribution, another possibly important variable, was also omitted, from scepticism about the quality of the available data.

The results of the multiple regression analysis were consistent with a quite orthodox view of the relation between social inputs and health status in developing countries. Of the seven variables considered, five showed favourable effects on infant mortality—physicians and other health workers per 1000 population, teachers in relation to school population (an index of educational quality), and proportion of the population with adequate water supply and excreta disposal (however only for the first and last was the relation statistically significant). The number of hospital beds per 1000 population was positively associated with IMR; this is consistent with the view that at a given level of the other variables, an emphasis on hospital care constitutes an inefficient use of health resources. More puzzling was the finding that per capita income was positively associated with infant mortality. It is not impossible to devise plausible explanations for this, but these are so various and conflicting that the safest conclusion seems to be the classic one—that more research is needed.

These results (which are taken from the second stage of the investigation, and differ somewhat from those in the publication cited) generally confirm the presumption that health is susceptible to manipulation through social inputs. But they do so essentially on a 'black box' basis—the mechanism joining inputs to output is in many cases obscure. It would be more satisfactory to develop models which specify the processes by which social inputs are linked to health outputs if the results are to serve for policy and planning.

Price and the demand for health services

To get beyond casual empiricism or 'black box' approaches, one needs testable models of the processes which connect development, health services, and health. It is natural for an economist to ask first whether any of the models which have already been developed in economics can be adapted to health. One of the simplest of these models is that which explains the quantity of a commodity demanded or consumed in terms of income and relative price. How far can one account for the relation between development and the consumption of health services in terms of income levels and the price of health care relative to other commodities on which consumers might spend their money? This question introduces a new subset of the relations between health and development; namely that of paying explicit attention to the price of health care.

While comparative international data on average incomes and some types of health service inputs are fairly easily available, data on total health care expenditure are less so (especially in developing countries), and data on comparative prices are almost non-existent. Hence, special interest attaches to the UN International Comparison Project (ICP) under which extensive price data are being collected as part of a study to establish a methodology for international income comparisons in terms of purchasing power. The most recent report covers sixteen developed and developing countries and provides income, consumption, and relative price data for 150 categories of commodities, including medical care as a whole and a number of sub-categories of health expenditure (Kravis, Heston, and Summers 1978). The report presents the results of regressing quantities consumed on relative price and per capita consumption (effectively, personal income) for the sixteen countries for 1970 and 1973. The regression coefficients (which can be treated as elasticities, since they are based on the logarithms of the variables) are, for medical care as a whole, -0.8 for price and 1.4 for income, with a value of R^2 of 0.96. In other words, one would expect a one per cent increase in the price of medical care to be associated with a decrease of 0.8 per cent in the quantity demanded, and a one per cent increase in the consumer's income to be associated with an increase in the quantity demanded of medical care of 1.4 per cent. Medical care, therefore, appears to behave as a moderately price-sensitive luxury good, and most of the international variation in its quantum per capita can be explained in price and income terms. When medical care is broken down into sub-categories (drugs, physicians' services, dentists' services, nurses' services, and hospital care), there is some variation in sensitivity to price changes (with drugs the most, and dentists' services the least, sensitive) and to incomes (with the elasticity for nurses' services being slightly less than unity). The proportion of variation explained is less than for medical care as a whole (R^2 from 0.76 to 0.92). But it remains true that, statistically speaking, the quantity of medical care 'consumed' per capita can be largely explained in terms of a quite conventional expenditure model using price and income as independent variables. The result is all the more impressive in that 'medical care' covered the whole field of health services, including much preventive work.

It can be argued, indeed, that the result is too clear-cut to be acceptable without further explanation. The normal interpretation of income and price elasticities depends on the theory of the choice of the individual consumer between goods available in the market. There are at least two reservations about applying this theory to the consumption of medical care. One is that the amount of medical care purchased is determined as much by the health professional as by the ultimate consumer. This, however, may apply less strongly to broad categories of medical care than to individual items, and also less to developing than to developed countries. The other difficulty is that, in some of the ICP countries, government expenditure accounts for a substantial part of medical care and of other categories of consumption also. One would expect this to weaken the kind of relation between income, price, and quantity of medical care which would be envisaged in a pure market situation.

There are at least two ways out of these difficulties, both of which require more elaborate modelling. One is to postulate decision patterns in the public sector which lead by a different path to the same results as in the private sector (e.g. the allocation of a fixed proportion of national income to government expenditure, and a fixed proportion of this in turn to health services, with the quantity of services provided thereby varying inversely with price). The other is to treat such items as 'drugs' and 'physicians' services' as inputs to a production process whose output is either health services or health, and which may be carried on by 'producers' at various levels, including that of the private household. This approach has affinities with the more general conception of the household as a producer of utilities (Becker 1965), a conception which has been fruitfully applied to the provision of health care, though only in relation to developed countries (Rosenzweig and Schultz 1980).

Interdisciplinary modelling

Most investigations of the connection between health services and health have been couched in broad terms, using aggregative indicators of the level of service (e.g. physicians per 1000 population) and of health (e.g. mortality rates). They have given little specific indication of the processes assumed to be at work, either on the side of expenditure or of disease control (with the partial exception of models of the costs and benefits of immunization). An important exception has been the model developed at the School of Public Health, University of Michigan (Grosse 1980).

This model was developed by professionals from a number of disciplines, including participants in the School's courses who had experience of particular developing countries. The essential elements in the model were estimates of mortality and morbidity at each age group from the main disease problems for typical populations; of the effects on these rates of providing particular patterns of health care and other social inputs such as sanitation and nutrition; and of the costs of the services provided. The estimates were arrived at partly by judgement and consensus, but they seem likely to be quite accurate enough for the purposes of the study, which were primarily to introduce health planners from developing countries to realistic quantitative planning techniques.

For a given population and total expenditure, the model permitted the calculation of the effect of different patterns of primary health care upon population coverage, and mortality and morbidity reduction by age group. While the study does not claim to be definitive, it does suggest at least one important conclusion; that approaches which concentrate resources in relatively intensive forms of health care (hospitals, health centres) may produce the greatest reduction in mortality and morbidity, though at the expense of limited population

coverage. It therefore identifies a possible conflict between two policy objectives
—mortality/morbidity reduction as against coverage—which has often been
assumed away in the literature on primary health care. It is hard to see how a
policy problem of this kind could have been usefully explored without the help of
a model of this type. It is worth drawing attention to the fact that the model was
specifically defined to permit the interaction of data from the side of both the
economist and the health professional, even though this no doubt meant simplifying
the picture as it might have been presented by either discipline for other purposes.

The economic consequences of malaria eradication

In the late 1940s, house spraying with DDT was introduced in a number of
developing countries as a means of controlling malaria, and in some (e.g. Sri
Lanka) was so successful at the time that the disease was considered eradicated.
This was a striking example of a major public health measure made possible by
technological advances and almost independent of the economic situation in the
countries where it was applied. Estimates indicated a major reduction in mortality
(Newman 1965) and, in spite of some contrary views, it is generally accepted
that this was due to the control of malaria (Gray 1974).

A fall in mortality implied an increase in the rate of population growth,
sufficient in the Sri Lankan case to have a significant effect on the balance
between this rate and the rate of growth of national income. It might be expected
that this would have both favourable and unfavourable effects on economic
development. On the one hand, the expansion of the labour force would increase
the productive capacity of the economy, subject to qualifications arising from
the presumption of a declining marginal productivity of labour. On the other
hand, the greater consumption demand, in both the public and private sectors,
would reduce the surplus available for investment, with consequences unfavourable to future production. The long-term effects of the decline in mortality
might conceivably be a reduction in economic growth and even in the per capita
resources available to health, offsetting the original improvement in national
health status. These implications were tested through a model of the Sri Lankan
economy incorporating an aggregate production function along with appropriate
demographic assumptions (Barlow 1968). The results appeared to confirm the
possibility that the favourable effects of malaria control might be self-negating
in the not too long run.

The conclusions of Barlow's study have been reduced in importance by Sri
Lanka's more recent economic vicissitudes, and also by the fact that malaria,
far from being eradicated, showed a sharp resurgence in the 1970s. But it has a
methodological importance as a demonstration of the possibilities of modelling
the interaction of development, health measures, and health status at the macroeconomic level.

Can health and nutrition interventions make a difference?

The ultimate test of hypotheses about the determinants of health in poor countries is the success or failure of interventions based on these hypotheses. This test has been least applied in the field of primary health care, a field which is expected to be of greatly increased importance in the next two decades. The above title is that of a study aimed at evaluating a number of primary care projects in developing countries (Gwatkin *et al*. 1980). The study was undertaken in the consciousness that a strong body of opinion existed which held that significant changes in the health of the general population of poor countries could only be brought about by broad social and economic changes which were outside the control of health authorities. The substantive conclusion of the study is that 'well-designed and carefully implemented interventions can reduce infant and child mortality by as much as one half within five years at a cost of below two per cent of per capita income'.

The study is also of interest because it shows the difficulties in the way of evaluating primary health care projects. Partly these spring from the inherent complexity of the relations involved, and the interactions of project components at the social and epidemiological levels. This difficulty is reinforced by the fact that successful projects often owe their existence to forceful leaders whose virtues are not replicable on a national scale. The other major source of difficulty is that the great majority of such projects are not designed for evaluation, except through day-to-day judgements of those who control them; it is rare to find provision for systematic collection of information, initially or during the course of the project, or for comparisons with control groups. The number of recorded projects in the primary health care field is in the hundreds, but the study found only ten with satisfactory provision for evaluation. This is a difficulty which can be reduced by better project and programme design. It is reasonable to expect that the evaluative component and the resources devoted to it should decline as one moves from the experimental project to the continuing programme, but in so complex and unpredictable a field it is likely that evaluation will be an important activity for the foreseeable future.

Conclusions

The relation between economic development, health services, and health has been presented here as one of forbidding complexity. Even so, there are a number of aspects of the relationship which have hardly been touched upon. For example, there has been no discussion of the relation between development and the international movement of goods and people, which is linked with health in several ways—the 'brain drain' of health professionals from poor to rich countries, the market situation of multinational drug manufacturers and others. Nor has the chapter attempted a complete account of the environmental effects of development on health—for example, the role of the agricultural use of DDT in promoting insecticide-resistance. The addition of such factors as these to the picture already outlined would reinforce the apparently pessimistic conclusion that there is not at the moment a comprehensive model of the processes at work which permits confident predictions of how a particular pattern of economic development and a particular level of health care will affect health in developing countries.

But one can also conclude more optimistically that the fragmentary models that do exist are already sufficient for certain important purposes. At the level of policy, there is sufficient evidence that at a given level of development, health can be improved through better health services and also through other social inputs. Even if it is not possible to arrive at universal statements of the relative importance of these inputs, they provide a checklist of relationships which can be explored for the purposes of national planning and project formulation, and which can be given a more specific and even quantitative form at that level. For such purposes, it is probably necessary to break down the concept of health into particular categories of diseases and of health problems. Eventually, the accumulation of data and the refinement of knowledge about particular problems should lead to the extension of the field over which reliable predictions and useful plans can be made.

This suggests certain priorities for further work. Sound physiological and epidemiological models are needed, since these are the foundations on which health economists must build; and these models should pay some attention to the problems of translating their conclusions into economic terms. From the economist's side, further work is required both on specific economic techniques and on national analyses of the relation between the resources devoted to social inputs and their 'output' in the form of health. Economists have a special responsibility for clarifying those calls on the health services, often treated with disrespect by health planners, which represent legitimate, even if subjective or even 'irrational', consumer demand rather than need as assessed by the health professions. Economists might also find it useful to search their repertoire for models applicable to the health sector outside conventional micro-economics and public finance—for example, in the fields of technical progress and innovation.

Finally, it can be argued that because of the complexity of the processes being dealt with, even when narrowed down to a single country or project, some space must always be left for learning by doing. It follows that the management of projects must make provision for continuous evaluation, even at some extra cost, and planners must be prepared to make use of the information thus generated. This suggests a closer integration of economists and economics into management than has been usual in the health sector.

REFERENCES

Abel-Smith, B. (1967). An international study of health expenditure and its relevance for health planning. *Publ. Hlth Pap. WHO* **32**.
— and Leiserson, A. (1978). Poverty, development and health policy. *Publ. Hlth Pap. WHO* **69**.
Barlow, R. (1968). *The economic effects of malaria eradication*. Research Series No. 15. Bureau of Public Health Economics, School of Public Health, University of Michigan.

Becker, G. S. (1965). A theory of the allocation of time. *Econ. J.* **75**, 493–517.

Cochrane, A. L., St. Leger, A. S., and Moore, F. (1978). Health service 'input' and mortality 'output' in developed countries. *J. Epidemiol. Community Hlth* **32** 200–5.

Cumper, G. E. (1980). *Resource requirement for achieving health for all by the year 2000.* Paper presented to Seminar on Costs and Financing Patterns of Primary Health Care. World Health Organization, Geneva.

— *Determinants of health levels in developing countries.* Research Studies Press, John Wiley and Sons. (In press.)

Gray, R. H. (1974). The decline of mortality in Ceylon and the demographic effects of malaria control. *Popul. Stud.* **28**, 205–30.

Grosse, R. N. (1980). Interrelation between health and population: observations derived from field experience. *Social Sci. Med.* **14C**, 99–120.

Gwatkin, D. R., Wilcox, J. R., and Wray, J. D. (1980). *Can health and nutrition interventions make a difference?* Overseas Development Council Monograph No. 13.

Kravis, I. B., Heston, A., and Summers, R., (1978). *International comparisons of real product and purchasing power.* Johns Hopkins University Press, Baltimore.

Newman, P. (1965). *Malaria eradication and population growth: with special reference to Ceylon and British Guiana.* Research Series No. 10, Bureau of Public Health Economics, School of Public Health, University of Michigan.

Preston, S. H. (1975). The changing relation between mortality and level of economic development. *Popul. Stud.* **29**, 231–48.

Rosenzweig, M. R. and Schultz, T. P. (1980). The behaviour of mothers as inputs to child health: the determinants of birthweight, gestation and rate of foetal growth. Paper presented to Conference on Economic Aspects of Health, National Bureau of Economic Research at Palo Alto.

St. Leger, A. S., Cochrane, A. L., and Moore, F. (1978). The anomaly that wouldn't go away. *Lancet* **8100**, 1153.

Author's note

The author would like to acknowledge his indebtedness to past and present colleagues at the University of the West Indies, the South-East Asia Regional Office and Headquarters Office of WHO, and the Ross Institute for the opportunity to discuss, with varying degrees of informality and acrimony, the ideas used in this chapter.

3

Health sector financing and expenditure surveys

Adrian Griffiths and Michael Mills

Introduction

This chapter consists of four sections. The first section outlines the use of economic information in health policy formation, and explains what health sector financing and expenditure surveys are, why they are needed, and how they may be used. The second section reviews the main stages in the development of such surveys since the late 1950s. The third section summarizes the main practical steps involved in their preparation and execution, and the emerging consensus about their most important conceptual and methodological aspects. The fourth section draws conclusions from the work done so far, and suggests key areas for future development.

Economic information and health policy

The State is now variously involved in financing, planning, and managing health services and other health-related activities in every country. Equal access to health care is widely accepted as a right, and recognized by the member states of the World Health Organization in the Declaration of Alma-Ata (WHO/UNICEF 1978), and its commitment to the target, 'Health for all by the year 2000'. At the same time, health care costs and expenditures in developed countries have been growing markedly faster than their gross national products in the last decade, as vividly described by the term 'health care cost explosion'.

If developing countries have not shown the same escalation in health sector spending as developed countries, it is because their resources do not allow it, but they face similar pressures. In addition, there is an increased awareness of the many factors which influence health, particularly activities which are not health services *per se*, but nevertheless are undertaken with a health-related intention. In consequence, health administrators have increasingly accepted the need not only for integrated health service planning, but also for integrated health *sector* planning, including non-service elements. Faced with laudable but desperately ambitious aims, the wider concept of the health sector, and increasing financial pressures, many countries are trying to reorient their health services and other health activities.

This situation is both of concern in health planning and a basic stimulus to it, particularly to efforts to achieve greater agreement between consumers, providers of services, and contributors of finance about the fundamental issues: health objectives and priorities; sources and allocation of resources; and effective and efficient methods of producing services. Ultimately this means paying greater attention to economic efficiency: to improve *allocative* efficiency—raising finance and allocating resources between different diseases, patients, geographical areas, and services so as to maximize the net benefit to society; and to improve *operational* efficiency—devising financing mechanisms and the least-costly methods of producing and delivering given health services to achieve required improvements in health status. Both these aims demand appropriate financing and payment mechanisms, to provide the necessary finance and facilitate the provision and use of services in the desired way, without imposing undue barriers to access, burdens of cost, or distortions in provision and use.

The objective of maximizing net benefit to society presupposes judgements about the relative social value of different outcomes. These judgements involve choices about:

(1) kinds of health improvement, e.g. reduced mortality versus reduced morbidity, or reductions in infectious versus chronic diseases;

(2) levels of improvement and their cost, e.g. total eradication of a disease at a particular cost versus partial reduction at a lesser cost;

(3) age, sex, and socioeconomic group to benefit, e.g. employed males aged 15-65 versus children under age 5 in poor families;

(4) geographical areas to benefit, e.g. region A versus region B; urban versus rural;

(5) incidence of costs and benefits between population groups, e.g. various types of 'equity' may be considered: *horizontal* equity—those with similar incomes pay equal amounts, or those with similar needs receive equal services; *vertical* equity—contributions are proportional to ability to pay, or services provided are proportional to need; and

(6) incidence of costs and benefits over time—cost and benefits may be closely linked in time, or benefits may be delayed for many years after the costs are incurred, perhaps to another generation.

Different financing structures have different deliberate and accidental cost and benefit redistribution effects which must be borne in mind.

Once such value judgements have been made, a number of different aspects of allocative and operational efficiency can be considered, for both the raising of revenue and the distribution of expenditures. These include:

(1) *Financial performance.* e.g. lotteries, one possible financing mechanism, are rather inefficient because of the high overhead costs of selling tickets and paying out of prizes; similarly for expenditures, the proportion of approved budgets actually spent may vary from one type of expenditure to another.

(2) *Social and political acceptability.* e.g. in financing there might be widespread evasion of unacceptable taxes; likewise, social and political resistance often

prevent the effective implementation of policies to reorient services from an urban, curative, and hospital basis to a rural, preventive, and ambulatory one.

(3) *Reliability*. e.g. certain taxes may be considered inefficient if there are large annual fluctuations in revenue; similarly, it may be inefficient to rely too much on foreign aid.

(4) *Flexibility*. e.g. costly investments in buildings, equipment, and highly-trained specialized staff have long lifetimes, and can tie up major expenditures in a relatively inflexible way.

(5) *Displacement*. e.g. a wealth tax might displace rather than complement charitable donations.

(6) *Impact on health and illness behaviour*. e.g. high tobacco and alcohol taxes might reduce associated health problems, whereas high user charges would reduce health service demands from the poor.

(7) *Effects on health service provision and functioning*. Financing and expenditure patterns can influence these in several ways: e.g. (i) the type of service provided—rural co-operatives might support village health workers, whereas insurance-funded fee-for-service payments might favour specialists and sophisticated diagnostic services; and (ii) service utilization—free publicly financed services are more likely to be used by the poor than are those financed by user charges.

(8) *Effects on the economy*. Health services and activities, even in developing countries, may account for up to six per cent of GDP, are major employers, and may also make significant demands on foreign exchange for training abroad and imports of equipment and drugs. Their financing and expenditures can, therefore, have important effects on the economy. These include (i) inflation, e.g. through high increases in staff pay; (ii) foreign exchange problems, e.g. through heavy foreign borrowing for development or large payments for imports; (iii) disincentives to investment, e.g. through high taxes on certain economic activities or sectors; (iv) opportunity costs, e.g. attraction of scarce manpower into the health professions at the expense of other sectors; and (v) improved economic productivity, e.g. through reducing preventable disability and death among the working population.

Financial data are the only convenient measure which enables all resources to be included in an overall view of the situation, and health planners and managers can only assess economic efficiency if they know about *total* spending from *all* sources. They need this information at the highest level of planning, to examine options and help establish priorities among health services and other health-related actions, particularly to weigh costs against effects or benefits. They also need it at successively lower levels, to decide how to adjust the system of organizing and financing services to achieve the objectives chosen; to assist operational management; and to evaluate policies during their implementation and provide feedback on the need for, and effectiveness of, corrective actions.

At present, in most developing countries, and indeed in many developed ones, health administrators tend to know only about the funds *they* control, and rarely about other health sector expenditures, such as expenditures by other government and state bodies, social security agencies, private insurance firms, charities, foreign aid, industry, and, last but not least, individuals.

In recent years, a few developing countries, organizations such as the World Health Organization, the World Bank, the American Public Health Association, the Sandoz Institute for Health and Socio-Economic Studies, and various academic institutions, have attempted to fill this gap in the knowledge through health sector financing and expenditure (HSFE) surveys. These have attempted to answer three basic questions.

(1) What is the total expenditure on the health sector?
(2) What are its sources and how much does each provide?
(3) On what is it spent?

While these survey efforts have often been made with minimal resources, and scarcely scratch the surface of the problem world-wide, they confirm for the countries covered, and suggest for others with similar health sector characteristics, that total expenditure may be two or three times higher than figures commonly quoted in official accounts. Differences of such magnitude are potentially of enormous importance in directing efforts to reorient health systems to a more effective and efficient pattern.

Why do countries not have this information? There are several major reasons for this seemingly surprising gap. First, there is a common tendency to regard the health sector as synonymous with health services, and a simultaneous but generally mistaken idea that spending by sources outside the main government health agencies is relatively unimportant. Secondly, in good bureaucratic tradition, ministries of health (or any other agency which might commission a health sector survey) tend to be reluctant to encroach on the organizational territory of other providers of finance and services, in the absence of a formal mandate to do so. Thirdly, an HSFE survey may be considered of limited use in so far as various providers of finance and services put their own independence of decision above the development of an integrated and co-operative policy. Finally, there has been a lack of a survey methodology that is relatively reliable, fast, and simple, and within the financial, technical, and logistic means of developing countries (WHO 1978). Fortunately, this situation is now changing, at least in terms of the methodology.

The development of health sector financing and expenditure surveys

In the space available it is not possible to review all the surveys so far done, or indeed to discuss in detail those included. The aim here is rather to describe the main stages in the development of such surveys, and the types of approach taken.

During the 1950s there was a growing interest in health service expenditures and costs, and national surveys began to be done, but they were concentrated in developed countries, and tended to cover only some sources of finance (ILO 1959; ISSA 1961).

The first systematic survey designed to obtain a relatively comprehensive accounting of all major sources of finance and expenditure on health services, and including *developing* countries, was a questionnaire-based survey by Abel-Smith for WHO (Abel-Smith 1963). The survey covered six countries, the developing ones being Sri Lanka and Chile. The results of this survey were so encouraging that a second, much larger study was designed, covering 29 countries, using a revised version of the questionnaire (Abel-Smith 1967). Of the countries surveyed, 21 were developing countries.

Since, as pointed out in the introduction to the first study, there was 'no international language of health service finance', both these studies attempted to define the various constituent components of the health services, to list the main sources of finance, and to lay down a standard classification of expenditures (including avoidance of double counting). This approach was an important methodological departure from previous attempts, which concentrated on the analysis of unstandardized existing data.

There were five important results. First, it was now possible to make valid international comparisons of health service financing and expenditure. These raised many fundamental questions about the differences between countries, and their significance in terms of the value for money achieved by different levels of spending, and by different systems of financing and strategies of expenditure. Secondly, a major impetus was given to repeat and extend such comparisons, and to improve the methodology (Simanis 1973; Kaser 1976; IEDES 1976; Poullier 1977; Abel-Smith and Maynard 1978; Bar and Richan 1979; Hauser and Koch 1980; Maxwell 1981). Though most of these comparative studies concentrated wholly on developed countries, they provided new and useful methodological insights of general relevance. Thirdly, these results were of considerable help in a parallel effort to define and classify health expenditures in the development of a uniform system of national accounts. Progress in this field is well illustrated in a review of Maxwell's study (Deering 1981). The reviewer, using only routine data on health expenditures from the *United Nations Statistical Year Book of National Accounts*, and the International Monetary Fund's *Government Financial Statistics Yearbook*, arrives at estimates of total health expenditure as a percentage of GDP identical or very close to those calculated with much more effort by Maxwell, but concedes that comparability problems arise when breakdowns of the total are attempted. Fourthly, developing countries were shown that total health service expenditures involved many more sources and services than had been previously accounted for, and represented a markedly higher percentage of GDP than hitherto believed. Fifthly, and very importantly, it was shown that such surveys could be done relatively quickly, with limited means, and should even be feasible in developing countries.

Given the above achievements, it was clear that a developing country could use the same type of approach to do more detailed studies, specially oriented to its own decision-making needs. Progress has been rather slower and less systematic than it might have been, but has accelerated since the mid-1970s. Many developing countries have sought better financial information to cope with the growing pressure of health sector expenditure on their always poor and now depressed economies. Others, having reached a certain level of development, have been anxious to examine the implications of introducing social security coverage of health services costs. Since 1978, the WHO target of 'Health for all by the year 2000' has added further impetus to such work, as countries consider how to reorient their services and to finance more primary care. In addition, more technical and financial help for such surveys has been forthcoming, albeit still extremely modest relative to the size of the task.

Some examples of the studies done since the late 1960s will illustrate the general trend. In 1969, Roemer published a review of the development of medical services under social security (Roemer 1969*a*), and followed this with a more specific review of Latin America (Roemer 1973). A joint WHO/ILO committee reported on the relationship between social security and personal health care (ILO/WHO 1971), and individual country analyses appeared for the Philippines (Sen 1975), for Rwanda (Nshimiyimana 1976), and for South Korea (Park 1977). In fact, these country studies were partial financing and expenditure surveys—they covered only some sources of finance and types of expenditures. But total coverage of all sources and expenditure is not mandatory, for one of the main objects of the methodology is precisely to tailor the scope of the survey to those policy questions of specific concern to the country.

The Korean study (1977) is a good example of policy relevance, for it was a baseline review of health needs and financing methods prior to the introduction of the new medical insurance programme in July 1977. The study focused particularly on the problems of deprived groups, such as rural populations, the poor, the self-employed, and employees of small firms. Its findings were extremely revealing. Private sources provided an enormous 87 per cent of overall health expenditure, which had grown very fast (threefold for public and fourfold for private spending between 1970 and 1975 alone). With such low public coverage, 40 per cent of people were estimated to receive no treatment when ill; and those who did often opted for self-medication or drug treatment (Western and traditional) largely from non-physicians (57 per cent of private spending), rather than more expensive care by doctors (33 per cent of private spending), or hospitals (only 8 per cent of private spending). This problem of high costs and inability to pay was confirmed by the geographical maldistribution of services; 83 per cent of doctors and 87 per cent of health facilities, but only 48 per cent of the population, were in urban areas. Doctors averaged only fifteen consultations a day, and hospital occupancy ranged from a very low 34 per cent in rural areas to only 61 per cent even in private urban hospitals.

At about the same time, another study was assisted by WHO in Bangladesh as part of a country health programming effort (Cumper, Chia, and Tarantale 1978). It differed from the Korean study in terms of its objectives, scope, data availability, and methods. However, it showed that, as in Korea, 87 per cent of (current) health expenditures came from private spending on curative services, with almost four-fifths of this going on drugs. Private urban curative spending alone slightly exceeded all government spending. Overall, per capita expenditure was about three times higher in urban than in rural areas, but the difference was only 2:1 for private spending per capita whereas it was 14:1 for government spending, half of which went on urban curative services (not allowing for the unknown but probably small percentage of rural residents treated in urban hospitals). This study also broke new ground in using data from sample epidemiological surveys to analyse expenditures between disease groups. It found that 57 per cent of total expenditures and 68 per cent of private expenditures went on only six disease groups (gastrointestinal diseases, skin diseases, influenza and upper respiratory infections, peptic ulcers and related conditions, nutritional diseases, and accidents).

Both these studies demonstrate vividly the enormous dependence on private expenditures, and the grossly misleading picture of health service spending provided by government expenditures, and even more by Ministry of Health expenditures, if taken alone. They also show that these very considerable amounts of private spending are spent largely on primary care and drugs, even though, to a large extent, only traditional healers and remedies are available. In other words, there already appears to be a substantial base for financing trained primary care workers and essential drugs, if they can be provided.

In 1976/77, the Sandoz Institute for Health and Socio-Economic Studies, in collaboration with WHO, started a small research programme to develop and test a simple, rapid, and cheap HSFE survey methodology for developing countries. The first result of this effort was a remarkably detailed and comprehensive survey done in Botswana in only nine weeks part-time, including the report itself, by the planning officer and two researchers (Ministry of Health of Botswana 1977). It found total expenditure to be considerably higher than previously thought, Pula 15.1 million or 5.3 per cent of GDP; that only 45.6 per cent of this came from government sources—central and local; that 33.2 per cent of total expenditure and a massive 93.2 per cent of capital expenditure came from aid; and that, though only a relatively low 16 per cent came from direct private spending, 42 per cent of this went on traditional healers and a further 32.1 per cent on drugs and medicines. The experience of this study provided the material for a detailed methodological report (Ministry of Health of Botswana 1978).

A parallel effort in the same programme examined the feasibility of using short-term foreign experts. Surveys were done in two French-speaking African countries, Senegal and Rwanda. In both cases data collection was completed within prearranged visits of only three weeks. The Senegal survey produced useful policy-related findings—e.g. major financing shortfalls against plans; declining Ministry of Health expenditures alongside increasing spending on military, police, and civil service health services; substantial regional inequalities in per capita spending (de la Grandville 1977). However, it encountered severe data problems which prevented even reliable estimates being made of several important sources of expenditure, notably private spending. The Rwanda study, though also unable to estimate direct private spending on private and traditional health services, showed once again that estimated expenditures (albeit incompletely measured) were much higher than those of the Ministry of Health. Of the estimated total of Rw.f. 2166 million, only 21.5 per cent came from government and another 14.8 per cent from individuals and industry, whereas 64 per cent came from aid (mainly bilateral and private) which, as in Botswana, provided virtually all the capital budget (Laurent 1978; Griffiths (1978*a*). This study showed, among other things, the value of complete information on expenditures for better co-ordination of aid, and to avoid gaps and duplications in allocations.

Confirmation of the feasibility of the approach was provided by the use of the Rwanda study methodology to do another survey of health service expenditures and sources in Togo (Sant-Anna 1981). This latter study underscores the differences between countries and the danger of generalizing, for it shows Togo to be much more self-sufficient in its health sector financing, with over half its health expenditure coming from government sources, over a quarter from individuals and industry, and under a fifth from foreign aid, most of it bilateral.

In 1978 the WHO held a study group meeting on the financing of health services, to review recent work and recommend future development. It concluded unequivocally that such surveys were useful, and that an appropriate methodology should be developed. Indeed, some efforts had already been made in this direction (Roemer 1969*b*; Zschock, Robertson, and Daly 1977).

In this context a second Botswana study was done in 1978/79 (Ministry of Health of Botswana 1979). It demonstrated that repeated studies were even more useful than single, one-off studies for they provide a basis for analysing trends and changes against policy. In addition, while improving on some aspects of the methodology developed in the first survey, it emphasized the importance of reliable estimation procedures. The second survey estimated total expenditure at Pula 39 million, almost two-and-a-half times the Pula 15.8 million estimate of the first study. A substantial part of this large difference arose from a wider definition of health expenditures in the second survey, and from real increases in expenditure, compounded by inflation, but different estimation procedures also played a significant role. For example, the second study, with more time and experience, and using multiple estimation methods, put private expenditures on traditional practitioners at Pula 3.3 million whereas the first survey, using only the Botswana Rural Income Distribution Survey, put it at only Pula 1 million. Soon after, an independent retrospective study of Ghanaian public health expenditure from 1967 to 1980 emphasized the large possible variation in expenditures from year to year, confirming the dangers of relying on one year's data in such circumstances (Brooks 1981).

The WHO continued its efforts to stimulate countries to undertake studies in this field with an interregional workshop on the financing of health services, aimed primarily at policy-makers (WHO 1980). However, the lack of a standard methodology suitable for field use remained a significant obstacle. Recognizing this, the Government of Botswana, aware of the value of its own two surveys, decided that this experience should be shared with its neighbours in the spirit of technical co-operation among developing countries. Accordingly, in collaboration with the Sandoz Institute, and with support from WHO and the American Public Health Association, a two-week training course in the methodology of HSFE surveys was organized in Gaborone at the end of 1980, for a small number of senior health service staff from Botswana, Lesotho, Malawi, Swaziland, and Zambia. This course enabled the present authors to prepare and test a set of training modules which have now been adapted into a practical manual for teaching and field use (Griffiths and Mills 1982). The following section reviews the main steps involved in an HSFE survey, and then discusses the most important conceptual and methodological points raised by such surveys.

Towards a methodology

The first question is who should initiate and authorize an HSFE survey? Clearly, each country will decide this for itself, but since the primary intention of such surveys is to provide a *complete* financial picture of the health sector, it is advantageous that they should, if possible, be done under the authority of the body or bodies chiefly concerned with the planning and provision of health services, usually the Ministry of Health in collaboration with other key bodies such as the social security agency or the Ministry of Planning. Furthermore, given the policy implications of such surveys and the wide ranging collaboration required from other bodies in carrying them out, it is important that authorization should be sought at top level, that is ministerial and chief officer level, and that what is to be done should be clear from the beginning.

The first technical step is the drafting of an outline survey proposal for approval. This should contain a preliminary statement of the proposed scope and objectives of the survey, together with an outline of the staff, budget, and programme of work envisaged. Once this is approved, a full-scale protocol can be prepared. The most important methodological elements of this protocol are: (1) the exact scope of the survey; (2) its specific objectives; (3) the sources of data to be consulted; (4) methods of data collection (including sequence and timetable); (5) methods of estimation, where appropriate; (6) records to be kept; (7) proposed analyses (including blank tables); and (8) the procedure for preparing and disseminating the report. Some of these elements are now explored below.

Definition of the health sector

It is essential to define precisely what services and activities comprise the health sector. The most widely used practical criterion is that health sector expenditures include capital and current expenditures on activities whose *primary* intention (regardless of effect) is to improve health. For example, expenditures on traditional medicines are included even if some are known to be ineffective, for the primary intent of the expenditure is nevertheless to improve health. More generally, such activities include health promotion and prevention, diagnosis, treatment, and care, and rehabilitation relating to illness, disability, or injury. They comprise both modern and traditional services; and expenditures on the education and training of health service staff, and on medical research, should also be included.

The usual ambulatory and hospital services are largely self-evident as categories to be included, but it must be remembered that such services may be provided by a wide range of bodies whose main business is not health, such as ministries of defence, interior, education, foreign affairs, and rural development; local government; industry; and private organizations. Also, supporting services such as transport and building services may be provided to the Ministry of Health by other ministries, and should be included.

Promotive and preventive services, such as health education, vaccination, and immunization, should clearly be counted, and there are less obvious, but similar, services, such as control of zoonotic diseases by the Ministry of Agriculture, some of which may well be done partly to protect human health. More difficult to decide upon are expenditures to improve water supply, nutrition, sanitation, environmental pollution, and occupational safety. A case can be made for including all of these expenditures (Ministry of Health of Botswana 1979)— for instance, it is arguable that improving health is the primary intent in providing clean water for domestic use, and safe sewage disposal. The inclusion of such items does however add huge amounts to health expenditures, and consequently completely overshadows the items more usually included. An additional criterion may therefore be required to avoid this dilemma. One which is both practical and widely accepted is that promotive and preventive expenditures should be included if their intention is to bring up to a minimum acceptable standard, individuals or populations with an identified health deficiency. For nutrition, this would mean including food supplements to meet diagnosed nutritional deficiencies but not mass food distribution programmes; and for water supply, sewerage and waste disposal services, only rural services, for instance to provide boreholes and pit latrines for populations with health problems arising from a lack of minimal facilities, but not major investments in sophisticated urban water and sewage systems.

As for education and training of health service staff and biomedical research, the key criterion distinguishing those expenditures which should be included is again whether their primary intention is to improve health. On this basis general education, as a prerequisite to specific medical and paramedical training, should not be included, nor should basic biological research (as opposed to medical and epidemiological research), for neither is sufficiently specific to health to warrant inclusion.

Scope and objectives

The three basic questions addressed by an HSFE survey have been stated in the first section, p. 46. At the practical level, however, the country's health problems, priorities, plans, and targets need to be carefully reviewed and a complete and specific set of objectives formulated for the survey, to ensure it meets the decision-making needs of policy-makers and managers, bearing in mind the availability or feasibility of obtaining the specific data envisaged. This should not, however, be interpreted as 'all or nothing', for as noted already some countries do have good information on some sources and expenditures, and may concentrate their survey effort on the gaps. Other countries, facing important policy decisions on particular sources or expenditures, or lacking the means to do a full survey, may decide to concentrate on a succession of partial surveys building up to a full picture. The only proviso to such an approach is that there should be a consistent overall design, as outlined above, to avoid methodological discrepancies.

During this preparatory process, systematic consultations are essential, on the one hand with users, to develop and agree on specific objectives, and on the other hand with the providers of data, to ensure that the objectives can be met from the data likely to be obtainable. Analyses of the surveys reviewed in the second section, p. 46 show that many of the difficulties encountered in collecting data, and ensuring that final tabulations met the decision-making needs of their intended users, arose largely from the absence or inadequacy of such preparatory consultations. Once agreed, the objectives can then be translated into a full set of proforma tables, so that all can see concretely how the final output will be presented *before* the survey begins. For example, if a breakdown by type of service is required, what service categories are wanted? Should hospital services be subdivided by types of hospital? Should in-patient and out-patient expenditures be distinguished?

Table 3.1 shows the main likely sources of health sector finance, and Table 3.2 shows the kinds of breakdowns which may be considered—though few surveys would be likely to provide them all. It is worth recalling here that the breakdowns will always show where money came from (sources of finance) against various classifications of how it was spent (categories of expenditures): that is, columns show how much finance each source provided, though some may have been transferred to another body to spend. In this respect, ministries are treated as sources, without identifying the sources which in turn provided the ministries' budgets. Likewise, insurance is treated as a source of finance without considering from where its revenue is derived.

The four main points to note are:

(1) The breakdowns chosen should provide a practical basis for evaluation of the main financial flows, and for decision-making.
(2) The usefulness of every breakdown proposed must be carefully weighed against the likely investment of time, effort, and money needed to obtain it

Table 3.1. *Main likely sources of finance*

I.   Government sources*

(a)   *Ministry of:*

(1) Health	(6) Rural Development	(11) Education
(2) Social Security	(7) Industry/Trade/	(12) Interior
(3) Local Government	Employment	(13) Foreign Affairs
(4) Transport and	(8) Mines	(14) Justice and Police
Communications	(9) Water Resources	(15) Defence
(5) Agriculture	(10) Public Works	

(b)   *Local government:*

(1) Regional	(3) Municipalities
(2) District	(4) Village councils

(c)   *Other public agencies:*

(1) Public utilities, providing water and/or sanitary services, etc.
(2) Nationalized industries
(3) Compulsory health insurance

II.   Religious organizations and domestic charities

(a)   Religious organizations/missions
(b)   Domestic charities and voluntary bodies

III. Private sources

(a)   *Private industry*

(b)   *Direct payments for:*

(1) In-patient and out-patient care in public and private hospitals, clinics, health posts, etc. (inc. fees paid to public services)
(2) Private practitioners
(3) Services abroad
(4) Private dental services
(5) Private ophthalmic services
(6) Other private health services, e.g. physiotherapy, nursing
(7) Private purchases of ethical and patent medicines, appliances and first-aid supplies
(8) Domestic water
(9) Transport required to use health services

IV.   External sources

(a)   *Foreign aid and technical co-operation:*†

(1) Bilateral governmental—by country of origin
(2) Multilateral governmental—by agency
(3) Private—by source

---

*This list is necessarily indicative for ministry titles and groupings vary from one country to another.
† Foreign aid may be in the forms of grants; loans; provision of subsidized or free staff, fellowships or supplies; or direct provision of health services.

TABLE 3.2. *Main types of breakdown of expenditures*

1. Type of service (e.g. hospitals, clinics, communicable disease control)
2. Diagnostic (main or important disease groups)
3. Geographical (e.g. region, district, urban/rural)
4. Population group (e.g. age, sex, social class)
5. Input category (e.g. staff, drugs, equipment)
6. Service provider
7. Combinations of the above (e.g. 1. and 3., 3. and 4.)
8. Comparison of any of the above against budgets
9. Time trends of any of the above (from repeated surveys)
10. Predictions of future situations based on trend projections or costing of anticipated developments

Note: Various types of unit cost can be calculated from the above breakdowns in association with other data (per unit of output, e.g. per in-patient case; per unit of effect, e.g. per unit of reduction in death rate).

(even if a particular breakdown is rejected as being too expensive, at least the information gap will have been explicitly recognized, and may be corrected by subsequent surveys or low cost changes in the routine information system).

(3) The summary tables should be kept to manageable proportions, so that the overall perspective of the situation is not lost in excessive detail; secondary breakdowns can always be provided to elaborate particular points.

(4) The main priority should be to present the findings of the survey in a policy and management oriented manner; methodological explanations should be limited to what the user needs in order to understand the results and to assess their reliability.

Data collection and tabulation

Once the blank tables have been prepared and agreed, the most convenient approach is to collect the data by source of finance, so that the final tables are built up systematically column by column. However, for some sources of finance, data collection may be complicated by the need to consult not only the different financing agencies and the final recipients, but also the intermediaries through which the finances are channelled. For example, foreign aid accounts are usually needed from all the various donors, but in order to find out exactly how the funds were spend, the accounts of intermediaries such as the Ministry of Health may also be needed, along with those of the final recipients such as missions or local government.

The order of tabulation depends on a number of factors. It is usually convenient to tabulate first those sources for which relatively complete figures are easily available and accessible, for instance government expenditures which are usually available from published accounts. This rule may be modified if such a source makes many transfer payments to other sources. In such cases, it may be hard to discover how such transfers were actually spent until the accounts for the recipient agencies have been examined, and it is often easier to postpone tabulation of the initial source of finance until this has been done. Also, particular groupings of sources may be wanted in the final tabulation, for instance all government sources or all foreign sources, and it may save restructuring the tables if they are tabulated in these groupings from the beginning.

Clearly, a major problem in HSFE surveys is *double-counting* of receipts or expenditures. If the prime objective is to know how much money is provided by each source, double-counting can be avoided by applying the rule: expenditures should be shown under the initial source of finance which provided the money, among the sources listed. Where one source (e.g. the Ministry of Health) transfers some of its funds to another agency (e.g. local government) which is also listed as a source of finance, or pays it for a service rendered, the amount involved should be shown in the column for the initial source of finance, that is the Ministry of Health and not local government. The same applies if a patient pays a mission hospital a fee for services received: the amount is shown in the column for direct private payments and not under missions.

Making estimates

Estimates of expenditures will be required in a number of situations. First, they will be required in those situations where the accounts are not in a suitable form to enable the required breakdowns to be made. This is often the case with Ministry of Health and other government accounts. Secondly, in multi-purpose activities the component of expenditure allocated to human health must be estimated, as in the case of zoonotic disease control by the veterinary department to protect both animal and human health.

Thirdly, estimates are required where the sources of finance or the providers of service, or both, keep few or no accounts, or are not prepared to make their accounts available. The main example of this is direct payment for health services by individuals. User fees paid to formal health services, such as public hospitals or clinics, are generally recorded in the accounts of these services, whereas direct payments by individuals to private practitioners (such as doctors, dentists, ophthalmologists, physiotherapists, nurses, and other paramedical staff) may not be well recorded by the recipients, who may in any case refuse to disclose them. Indigenous practitioners are extremely unlikely to keep such accounts, and are often largely paid in kind.

A variety of methods exist to estimate these expenditures. They include: (1) special surveys and interviews with samples of the various service providers concerned; (2) adaptation of data from more general income studies, such as rural income surveys; (3) analyses of tax records relating to the various provider groups; (4) estimates based on household expenditure surveys; (5) estimates based on health insurance accounts; (6) macro estimates of revenue or expenditure from national income accounts; (7) costings of prescription statistics; and (8) trade and production statistics for commodities such as drugs and appliances.

Final tabulations and evaluation

As already indicated, the final tabulations depend on the objectives set for the survey at the beginning; and the results should be evaluated in terms of their consistency with established health policy, both tables and findings being presented in a policy- and decision-oriented manner. To illustrate these points, tables have been drawn from the HSFE manual (Griffiths and Mills 1982). They are based on real data from the Republic of Botswana, but have been amplified and in some cases supplemented by imaginary data to emphasize certain points. The conclusions drawn should not, therefore, be taken as applying to Botswana.

Table 3.3 illustrates a basic breakdown of current expenditures, from twelve sources of finance broken down into 28 expenditure categories, based on types of service. Analysis of each column shows how each source spent its money, and analysis of each line shows how each type of service was financed. For example, the Ministry of Health column shows that it spent Pula 1 000 000 (14 per cent of its total current expenditure) on the national referral teaching hospital; while the row for general hospitals shows that the Ministry of Health provided Pula 2 960 000 (50 per cent of the total) for the current financing of general hospitals.

Some of the possible breakdowns which might then be required have already been listed in Table 3.2. Table 3.4 illustrates one of these—estimated current expenditures on primary health care (PHC). The procedure used to derive this was relatively simple, and in some cases somewhat arbitrary, but it provides a reasonably accurate, yet practical, estimate. Each of the expenditure categories in Table 3.3 was examined to see whether or not the services concerned provided PHC and, if only partially, what proportion it represented of their expenditures. (Such proportions can sometimes be calculated directly from the accounts of the various services, but may also require information on the characteristics of the services and their utilization as in the case of hospital out-patient services which may be primary, secondary or even tertiary.) This analysis showed that PHC accounted for 20 per cent of general hospital and central laboratory services (categories 2 and 22); 50 per cent of private dentistry, other private services, and transport expenditure (categories 12, 14, 25); and all of the various ambulatory service expenditures (categories 7-11), retail sales of drugs and dressings (category 13), and the various basic health and preventive programmes (categories 15-21).

The illustrative data in Table 3.4 show that total current expenditure on PHC amounts to just over Pula 15 million which represents a substantial 58.9 per cent of total current expenditure. They also show, however, that the biggest source of finance is not the Ministry of Health (8.8 per cent) or even all government sources combined (38.7 per cent), but direct private payments by individuals (47.7 per cent). Furthermore, Pula 4.25 million or almost 60 per cent of these private expenditures went to indigenous practitioners, whereas all the PHC services provided by the various clinics, health posts, and private practitioners

TABLE 3.3. *Health sector current expenditures*

	1 Ministry of Health	2 Other ministries	3 Local government	4 Other state bodies	5 Missions	6 Industry	7 Local voluntary bodies	8 Direct private payments by individuals	9 Insurance	10 Self-help other private sources	11 Foreign aid — official	12 Foreign aid — private	Total
1. Teaching/national referral hospital	1 000 000	60 000						165 000	100 000		24 000		1 349 000
2. General hospitals	2 960 000	76 000			720 000	800 000		745 000		480 000	84 000		5 865 000
3. Long stay hospital	450 000	12 000						55 000					517 000
4. Mental hospital	400 000	8000						55 000					463 000
5. Other institutions (specify)						50 000	15 000	500 000					565 000
6. Services abroad													
7. Health centres/clinics with medical staff			708 000					32 000			60 000	100 000	900 000
8. Health centres/clinics with paramedical/nursing staff			690 000				16 000	57 000		8000		16 000	787 000
9. Health posts with community health workers only			150 000					35 000					185 000
10. Private practitioners								300 000	50 000				350 000
11. Indigenous practitioners								4 250 000					4 250 000
12. Private dental services								50 000	20 000				70 000
13. Retail outlets (drugs/dressings)								1 200 000					1 200 000
14. Other private services (specify)								40 000					40 000
15. Communicable disease control	200 000	450 000											650 000
16. Domestic water supplies		1 500 000						1 100 000					2 600 000
17. Sanitation programmes	160 000	200 000	127 000			100 000					15 000		602 000
18. Nutrition programmes	50 000	100 000					10 000				1 000 000	20 000	1 180 000
19. Health education programmes	100 000												100 000
20. Occupational health programmes	30 000					50 000							80 000
21. Other programmes (specify)	60 000										100 000		160 000
22. Central laboratory service	300 000												300 000
23. Travelling and transport	140 000	750 000	350 000		30 000	90 000		10 000		20 000			1 390 000
24. Headquarters administration	650 000	4000	145 000		50 000				50 000				899 000
25. Training —doctors, dentists		30 000									160 000		190 000
26. Training —other health staff	650 000	40 000									150 000		840 000
27. Medical research													
28. Other services (specify)													
Transfer (miscellaneous)													
Total	7 150 000	3 230 000	2 170 000		800 000	1 090 000	41 000	8 594 000	220 000	508 000	1 593 000	136 000	25 532 000

TABLE 3.4. Expenditures on primary health care (current)

	1 Ministry of Health	2 Other ministries	3 Local government	4 Other state bodies	5 Missions	6 Industry	7 Local voluntary bodies	8 Direct private payments by individuals	9 Insurance	10 Self-help other private sources	11 Foreign aid —official	12 Foreign aid —private	Total
1. Teaching/national referral hospital	592 000	—	—	—	144 000	160 000	—	149 000	—	96 000	16 800	—	1 173 000
2. General hospitals	—	15 200	—	—	—	—	—	—	—	—	—	—	—
3. Long stay hospital	—	—	—	—	—	—	—	—	—	—	—	—	—
4. Mental hospital	—	—	—	—	—	—	—	—	—	—	—	—	—
5. Other institutions (specify)	—	—	—	—	—	—	—	—	—	—	—	—	—
6. Services abroad	—	—	—	—	—	—	—	—	—	—	—	—	—
7. Health centres/clinics with medical staff	—	—	708 000	—	—	—	—	32 000	—	—	60 000	100 000	900 000
8. Health centres/clinics with paramedical/nursing staff	—	—	690 000	—	—	—	—	57 000	—	8 000	16 000	16 000	787 000
9. Health posts with community health workers only	—	—	150 000	—	—	—	16 000	35 000	—	—	—	—	185 000
10. Private practitioners	—	—	—	—	—	—	—	300 000	50 000	—	—	—	350 000
11. Indigenous health practitioners	—	—	—	—	—	—	—	4 250 000	—	—	—	—	4 250 000
12. Private dental services	—	—	—	—	—	—	—	25 000	10 000	—	—	—	35 000
13. Retail outlets (drugs/dressings)	—	—	—	—	—	—	—	1 200 000	—	—	—	—	1 200 000
14. Other private services (specify)	—	450 000	—	—	—	—	—	20 000	—	—	—	—	20 000
15. Communicable disease control	200 000	1 500 000	—	—	—	—	—	—	—	—	—	—	650 000
16. Domestic water supplies	—	—	—	—	—	—	—	1 100 000	—	—	—	—	2 600 000
17. Sanitation programmes	160 000	200 000	127 000	—	—	100 000	—	—	—	—	15 000	—	602 000
18. Nutrition programmes	50 000	100 000	—	—	—	10 000	—	—	—	—	1 000 000	20 000	1 180 000
19. Health education programmes	100 000	—	—	—	—	—	—	—	—	—	—	—	100 000
20. Occupational health programmes	30 000	—	—	—	—	50 000	—	—	—	—	—	—	80 000
21. Other programmes (specify)	60 000	—	—	—	15 000	—	—	—	—	—	100 000	—	160 000
22. Central laboratory service	60 000	375 000	175 000	—	—	—	—	—	—	10 000	15 000	—	625 000
23. Travelling and transport	70 000	—	—	—	—	45 000	—	5000	—	—	—	—	130 000
24. Headquarters administration	—	—	—	—	—	—	—	—	—	—	—	—	—
25. Training—doctors, dentists	—	—	—	—	—	—	—	—	—	—	—	—	—
26. Training—other health staff	—	—	—	—	—	—	—	—	*	—	—	—	—
27. Medical research	—	—	—	—	—	—	—	—	—	—	—	—	—
28. Other services (specify)	—	—	—	—	—	—	—	—	—	—	—	—	—
Total	1 322 000	2 640 200	1 850 000	—	159 000	365 000	16 000	7 173 000	60 000	114 000	1 191 800	136 000	15 027 000
(%)	8.80	17.57	12.31	—	1.06	2.43	0.11	47.73	0.40	0.76	7.93	0.91	100

covered by expenditure categories 7-10 accounted for only Pula 2.2 million. In other words, on the basis of this data it can be concluded that there is substantial room for tapping existing financial resources to extend formal rural PHC services—if appropriate mechanisms can be found. For example if a health post costs Pula 3700 a year to run, just 25 per cent of the private direct expenditures would support 287 such posts, which would cover over 140 000 people if each on average served a population of 500.

It is not the intention here to embark upon a detailed interpretation of the illustrative data in Tables 3.3 and 3.4. However, a brief example will show the importance both of having a complete financial picture in deciding policy, and of a precise, preferably quantified, formulation of what is decided. Suppose the policy document merely states that priority in current expenditure should be given to PHC. The first requirement is to have a precise definition of the expenditures to be included under PHC. For illustrative purposes, assume the calculations used to derive Table 3.4 are acceptable. (Of course, other assumptions might have been made, for instance that no hospital services belong in PHC, in which case total PHC expenditure would have been Pula 1 173 000 less.) If the Ministry of Health examines only its own expenditures (column one in Tables 3.3 and 3.4), it would conclude that only 18.5 per cent (Pula 1 322 000/ 7 150 000) of its current expenditure went on PHC, and might decide that this was unacceptably low. However, if it extends its analyses to other government sources it would find that the percentages of current expenditure allocated to PHC are: other ministries, 81.7 per cent; local government, 85.3 per cent; and all government sources, 46.3 per cent. If the analyses are extended to all sources of finance the percentage allocated to PHC is found to be 58.9 per cent. Clearly, therefore, possession of expenditure data for all financing sources substantially changes the policy conclusions and highlights the importance of detailed, preferably quantified, policy statements.

Conclusions and future developments

It is evident from the experience described above that a simple, standard survey methodology, especially when allied with standardized national accounts, can provide valuable information quickly and cheaply for health policy and management decisions in developing countries. Many criteria may be applied to evaluate management information (Griffiths 1978b) such as that provided by these surveys. However, there is only one ultimate justification for them, that the information they provide can be and actually is used to improve the performance of health services and activities. Their development is not an end in itself. Measured against this criterion, the results of previous HSFE surveys have been disappointing.

There are several reasons for this lack of success. Some surveys have been prompted and/or done by outsiders without adequate consultation with the potential users beforehand, and without proper feedback of the results in an appropriate form afterwards. In others, crude methodology, heroic estimates and incomplete data have failed to inspire confidence in the results. In many countries, policies have been formulated in such general terms that it has proved impossible to assess survey results against them and, in any case, health service capacity to absorb and use the information has often been severely limited, particularly in the poorest countries. Vested interests and social pressures have also prevailed over efforts to implement change. Finally, many important health service inputs, such as professional staff and complex buildings, often involve long lead-times and high costs. Furthermore, once produced they last a long time. For both these reasons they are hard to change quickly, and changes underway may not be easily discernible in the short run.

A number of developments in health sector financing and expenditure surveys are now needed:

(1) to test, refine, adapt, and extend the methodology to systems with different patterns of organization and financing, for instance to those with predominantly social security or insurance-based financing; to large countries where the logistical problems of surveys may be considerable; and, to 'federal' countries where there are more transfers between levels of government;

(2) to integrate this kind of analytical work into the overall context of routine health planning and management;

(3) to improve the detailed specification of health policy statements so that they can be used to interpret and evaluate the findings of HSFE surveys;

(4) to adapt the routine information system to provide the necessary data with minimum extra work;

(5) to mobilize this kind of approach in pursuit of the objective 'Health for all by the year 2000', particularly to help reorientate health services and find new sources and mechanisms for financing primary care; several of the studies quoted above found that considerable private spending by individuals already exists—knowing its magnitude and the ways in which it is distributed, attempts could be made to harness it more effectively; and

(6) to use HSFE survey data to co-ordinate and improve the efficiency and effectiveness of key development resources such as foreign aid allocations.

REFERENCES

Abel-Smith, B. (1963). Paying for health services: a study of the costs and sources of finance in six countries. *Publ. Hlth Pap. WHO* **17**.
— (1967). An international study of health expenditure and its relevance for health planning. *Publ. Hlth Pap. WHO* **32**.
— and Maynard, A. (1978). *The organisation, financing and cost of health care in the European communities* (SEC (78)3862). Commission of the European Communities, Brussels.
Bar, A. M. and Richan, H. (1979). Die Entwicklung der Staatlichen Aufwendungen und der Beschäftigtenzahl in Gesundheits und Sozialwesen— Ausdruck der Fürsorge des Sozialitischen Staates, [The development of national expenditure and employment in the health and social sector— health care in the socialist states.] *Z. ges. Hyg.* **25**, 772-5.

Brooks, R. G. (1981). Ghana's health expenditures 1966–1980: A commentary. Strathclyde Discussion Paper in Economics 81/1. Department of Economics, University of Strathclyde, Glasgow.

Cumper, G. E., Chia, M., and Tarantale, D. (1978). Expenditure on health in Bangladesh 1976. Annex 1 of WHO (1978).

Deering, J. A. (1981). Book review. *Health Affairs* 1, 105–17.

de la Grandville, O. (1977). Health expenditure in Senegal and its financing. Background paper for WHO Study Group on Financing of Health Services.

Griffiths, D. A. T. (1978a). The financing of health services in Rwanda (English summary of Laurent (1978)). (Mimeo.) Sandoz Institute for Health and Socio-Economic Studies, Geneva.

—— (1978b). Evaluating information for management. *Hospital and Health Services Review* August, pp. 259–63.

—— and Mills, M. H. (1982). *Health sector financing and expenditure surveys in developing countries: A methodological manual.* Third World Series, Sandoz Institute for Health and Socio-Economic Studies and the Ministry of Health, Republic of Botswana.

Hauser, H. and Koch, H. (1980). Health economic expenditure and its financing: An international survey on cost sharing. In *Proceedings of the international seminar on cost sharing* (ed. B. Horisberger *et al.*) Martin Robertson, London.

IEDES (Institut d'Étude du Développement Économique et Social) (1976). Le financement du systéme sanitaire dans 14 états Africains et Malgâches 1970–1974. Institut d'Étude du Développement Économique et Social, Paris.

ILO (International Labour Office) (1959). *The cost of medical care.* International Labour Office, Geneva.

ILO/WHO (International Labour Office/World Health Organization) (1971). Personal health care and social security: report of a joint ILO/WHO Committee. *Tech. Rep. Ser. Wld Hlth Org.* **480.**

ISSA (International Social Security Association) (1961). *Volume and cost of sickness benefits in kind and cash.* International Social Security Association, Geneva.

Kaser, M. (1976). *Health care in the Soviet Union and Eastern Europe.* Croom Helm, London.

Laurent, A. (1978). Le Financement des Services de Santé au Rwanda. Sandoz Institute for Health and Socio-Economic Studies, in collaboration with WHO.

Maxwell, R. J. (1981). *Health and wealth: An international study of health care spending.* Lexington Books, Lexington, Mass., for the Sandoz Institute for Health and Socio-Economic Studies.

Ministry of Health of Botswana (Kam, P. M., Malotle, M. P., and Raditladi, M. D.) (1977). A country case study: financing of health services in Botswana. (Mimeo.) Ministry of Health, Gaborone, Republic of Botswana.

—— (Kam, M. P.) (1978). Methodology for the survey and analysis of health financing and expenditure in Botswana. (Mimeo.) Ministry of Health, Republic of Botswana.

—— (Mills, M. H., Breutner, C., and Kgathi, L.) (1979). The financing of health services in Botswana: second study 1979. (Mimeo.) Ministry of Health, Republic of Botswana.

Nshimiyimana, F. (1976). Étude sur l'etablissement d'un régime d'assurance-maladie au Rwanda, Kigali: caisse sociale du Rwanda. (Mimeo.)

Park, C. K. (1977). *Financing health care in Korea.* Korea Development Institute, Seoul.

Poullier, J. -P. (1977). *Public expenditure on health*. OECD studies in Resource Allocation No. 4. Organization for Economic Co-operation and Development, Paris.

Roemer, M. I. (1969*a*). *The organisation of medical services under social security*. International Labour Office, Geneva.

— (1969*b*). Socioeconomic aspects of health services research in Colombia: a methodology for research. A consultation report prepared on the invitation of the Pan American Health Organization and the Milbank Memorial Fund. (Mimeo.) Washington.

— (1973). *Development of medical services under social security in Latin America*. International Labour Office, Geneva.

Sant-Anna, M. (1981). Le financement des dépenses de santé au Togo. Memoire de licence en Science Hospitalière en Administration et Gestion des Institutions Hospitalières et Médico-sociales, École de Santé Publique, Faculté de Médicine et de Pharmacie, Université Libre de Bruxelles.

Sen, P. (1975). Financing Medical Care Insurance in the Philippines. *Int. Social Security Rev.* 2, 139–50.

Simanis, J. G. (1973). Medical care expenditures in seven countries. *Social Security Bull.* March.

WHO (World Health Organization) (1978). Financing of health services. *Tech. Rep. Ser. Wld Hlth Org.* **625**.

— (1980). Financing of Health Services. Proceedings of a WHO interregional workshop, Mexico, 26–30 November 1979, SHS/SPM/80.3. World Health Organization, Geneva.

WHO/UNICEF (World Health Organization/United Nations International Children's Emergency Fund) (1978). Report of the International Conference on Primary Health Care, 6–12 September 1978, Alma-Ata, USSR, ICPHC/ALA 78.10. World Health Organization and United Nations Children's Fund.

Zschock, D. K., Robertson, R. L., and Daly, J. A. (1977). *How to study health sector financing in developing countries*. A manual prepared for the Office of International Health, Department of Health, Education and Welfare, Washington.

Authors' note

This chapter, particularly the third section, draws heavily on work undertaken by the authors as co-organizers of a course held in Gaborone at the end of 1980 on the methodology of HSFE surveys. This course was run by the Government of Botswana and the Sandoz Institute for Health and Socio-Economic Studies, with the sponsorship of, and attendance by staff from WHO and the American Public Health Association. The authors are particularly grateful to Dr David Sebina, Permanent Secretary of the Ministry of Health of Botswana, who initiated this course and supported it through to fruition; and to the senior health service staff who attended from Botswana, Lesotho, Malawi, Swaziland, and Zambia, who so ably helped to test and improve the survey material.

The views and interpretations in this chapter are those of the authors and should not be attributed to the Sandoz Institute, the World Bank, or any of the participants on the course in Botswana.

4

Economic aspects of health insurance

Anne Mills

The significance of health insurance

Many governments in developing countries, faced with an increasingly hostile economic environment, growing popular (and international) demands for the extension of health services, and increasing pressure on government budgets, are seeking ways of financing the expansion of their health care systems that do not depend upon the availability of general tax revenues. A few countries are considering increased reliance on private mechanisms; others are looking for collective mechanisms at the community, regional, or national level. In both cases, countries will wish to consider whether or not health insurance is a suitable source of additional resources for health care.

The reasons for choosing health insurance systems as the subject of this chapter are fivefold. First, since health insurance may be organized on either a private or public basis, it offers the opportunity to review some of the arguments on whether health care should be financed and/or provided via private markets or public agencies. The development of a government-regulated, financed, and even publicly provided health service is an implicit goal in the health policy of many developing countries, especially in Africa. Why should there be this emphasis on the direct involvement of government? In countries with an essentially capitalist mode of production, sectors equally vital to human survival such as food production and consumption have been left largely to private markets to organize. Nor do arguments that health care is unusual—because demand for health care is irregular and unpredictable, care can be lengthy and expensive, and illness has a high cost in terms of lost productive capacity—of themselves support government intervention, but may simply suggest a potential role of some form of health insurance, to protect the individual and family against uncertain events.

The issues of why governments should intervene in the health care market and whether on *a priori* grounds health care is most efficiently organized by the private or public sector have intrigued economists and produced a considerable theoretical debate (Culyer 1972, 1976). The debate was inconclusive, but only in the sense that it proved not possible, on theoretical grounds, to demonstrate one system of organization to be more efficient than another. What matters are the objectives a country seeks to achieve through its health system and the extent to which the health system achieves these objectives in practice.

The second reason for focusing on health insurance in this chapter is that the potential for expanding the health sector through increased government finance is likely to be very limited in many developing countries, even if the initial cost is relieved by external aid. The tax base is often very narrow, consisting largely of indirect taxes such as customs duties, and receipts from direct taxes such as income tax are typically low. Some form of health insurance, requiring contributions by individuals and/or employers, often appears attractive to a health sector starved of funds and doubtful of getting revenue from other quarters.

Thirdly, health insurance schemes are already widespread in the developing world. A recent review showed that more than half of all low and middle income developing countries have some form of medical insurance as part of their social security system (Zschock 1982). They include all Latin American countries and a number of African and Asian countries. Table 4.1 indicates that it is not only the richest of these countries that have such health insurance.

TABLE 4.1. *Medical care under social security: low and middle income countries*

Per capita income (1978)	Number of countries	Number with any type of social security programme	Number with medical care component
Below $500	47	33	19
$500–$1000	18	14	11
$1000–$2000	16	15	12
Above $2000	9	7	6
Total	90	69	48

Source: Zschock 1982

These figures are, however, somewhat misleading, for only in a few Latin American countries do contributions constitute a significant proportion of total medical care expenditures. Moreover, health insurance typically covers a small proportion of the population, usually the higher wage earners in the modern sector of the economy. Insurance systems in developing countries have therefore catered mainly for the urban elite.

Such characteristics have contributed to considerable controversy on the desirability of social insurance systems of medical care in developing countries, on their impact on the health services received by other sectors of society, and on their impact on the health of the whole population. This controversy introduces a fourth reason for examining health insurance. The protagonists of social insurance argue that it taps money which otherwise would not be spent on health care; provides a stable source of revenue for the health sector; does not reduce the funds available for Ministry of Health services; improves the health of those workers most vital for a country's growth; and, when it provides its own facilities, uses funds more efficiently than the private sector which might grow rapidly in the absence of insurance (Roemer 1971). Opponents argue that insurance systems are inequitable in practice: they benefit a small elite but impose costs on the rest of society because they absorb scarce staff, promote curative, high-cost care and inappropriate medical education, and are often subsidized by taxes which may weigh most heavily on the poorer sections of the population (Abel-Smith 1978). Health insurance has thus been criticized as representing a Western model whose transfer to the developing world is inappropriate.

It is certainly true that health insurance has been and still is an important source of finance in developed countries, and for that reason is worthy of scrutiny to see whether useful lessons can be learnt from their experience. The United States is exceptional in having a very extensive, privately organized (though often non-profit making) health system based on private insurance. Most European countries, such as France, Germany, and The Netherlands, have almost total social insurance coverage, though with considerable government regulation and financial support for the premiums of the elderly, unemployed, and indigent (Blanpain 1978). Only in a few countries, such as the United Kingdom and Sweden and more recently Italy and Denmark, has the insurance principle been largely abandoned in favour of a national health service funded from general tax revenues. Yet even in the United Kingdom, traditionally seen as the birth-place of a 'socialized' health system, there has been renewed interest of late in private insurance as a means of increasing the resources available for health care, thus reviving the controversy on the merits of insurance systems (Maynard 1979*b*; Abel-Smith 1981; Torrens 1982).

The objectives of this chapter are to set out the aims and role of health insurance systems; to examine the case for health insurance in developing countries; and to look at the way schemes are operating in practice in both rich and poor countries. The chapter first attempts to clarify the nature of health insurance and the various forms it can take. The next section examines these various forms of health insurance system, concentrating on their economic efficiency and equity implications. Before examining the experience of developing countries, the United States system is analysed partly to provide an object lesson in how not to do it, but also to note some of the recent innovations in decentralized forms of provision that may offer promise of a more efficient and cost-effective American health care system. The operation of health insurance systems in developing countries is then studied, important issues and problems are identified and possible solutions suggested. The chapter ends with some conclusions on the potential of the insurance mechanism as a source of funds for health care in developing countries, and provides a list of criteria which can be used to evaluate existing or prospective health insurance systems.

What is health insurance?

Insurance provides the means by which risks, or uncertain events, are shared between many people. Premiums are paid to an insurance institution which compensates any insured victim of the event for any financial loss resulting from the event. Insurance therefore helps to lessen and spread risks, and it relies on the fact that what is unpredictable for an individual is highly predictable for a large number of individuals. It follows that for insurance to be feasible, there must be enough individuals insured to spread the risks widely, and the uncertain events must be relatively independent of each other. That is, the principle is one of insurance based on probabilities, not one of prepayment for known future events; though in practice, a prepayment element for health care exists since certain types of utilization are highly predictable. For a health insurance scheme to be cost covering, the level of its premiums needs to be related to the statistical frequency with which the population covered requires care, and to the average cost of claims, plus an allowance for administrative costs and a profit margin (for commercial institutions).

Insurance inevitably has redistributive consequences, their nature and magnitude depending on the financing of the schemes and the way in which premiums are assessed. Because the occurrence of the event being insured against is uncertain, some participants will draw out more than they pay in, thus resulting in redistribution from the healthy to the sick. Other distributive effects will depend, as discussed below, on whether the insurance is organized privately or through collective mechanisms, and on the method of distributing the costs over the population.

Health insurance can be financed and organized in a variety of different ways. It can be purchased by an individual or group through the private market, from either profit or non-profit firms, and under these circumstances is conventionally termed private or voluntary health insurance. Health care itself would usually be delivered by independent providers, but sometimes by facilities owned by the insurer.

The level of an individual's premium would be based on the actuarially-determined likelihood of illness of that individual. In contrast, group insurance is often based on a firm or co-operative, and the premiums related to the risk of the group of employees *in toto*, not of individuals. All subscribers will pay similar premiums (except for adjustments for the size of family covered), and such insurance may well be made compulsory by the firm to prevent low risk or high income employees opting out. In some countries (for instance the United States and Australia) there are examples of the imposition of 'community rating' on private insurers; that is, within a given geographical area, premiums are not permitted to vary according to health risk or occupation (Feldstein 1979; Scotton 1974). Premiums are often paid at least in part by employers, health insurance being considered a fringe benefit, though labour legislation making it compulsory for employers to provide their workers with some form of medical care is increasingly being introduced in developing countries (WHO 1978).

An individual's demand for private health insurance will be determined by factors such as the price of insurance, that is the premiums to be paid; the individual's assessment of the probability of loss (especially financial) resulting from illness; the likely magnitude of that loss; his income; and most especially, the degree to which he is risk averse (Feldstein 1979). Considerable attention has been given to whether or not a private market in health insurance would necessarily lead to the optimal amount of insurance, or whether there would be people who are either over-insured (for instance because the opportunity cost to them of insurance has been reduced by employer contributions or tax-offset arrangements) or under-insured (for instance because policies are not offered to low income groups or high risks) (Maynard 1979*b*). In any case, a section of the population will lack either the purchasing power or the will to obtain the amount of cover society considers they ought to have, and thus would not be adequately protected under a private market system of insurance unless they were given special assistance.

Health insurance organized by the state or by a public body is usually termed social insurance, social security, or sometimes compulsory health insurance. Social insurance schemes usually incorporate income maintenance measures as well, are compulsory for all individuals falling within the schemes and are seen as a source of not only individual but also community welfare. The conventional funding source for social insurance consists of payroll taxes levied on workers and employers, often supplemented by user fees and by government contributions from tax revenues. If the scheme is self-financing the total contributions collected should be actuarially determined on the basis of the probability of the events insured against occurring, but contributions from workers and employers can be either flat rate, or earnings-related (usually within certain prescribed limits). Some countries have a single social insurance fund; others have multiple sickness funds, often organized on a firm or industry basis.

It is important to note that state involvement in health care financing, through the regulation of private insurance or the organization of social insurance, does not of itself demand state involvement in the provision of care. Thus it is important to distinguish between systems *providing* health services and systems *paying* for health services which are provided by commercial, voluntary, or non-profit agencies, institutions, and personnel (Kohn 1980). The state or a parastatal organization may operate both an insurance fund and health care institutions for the insured; it may operate institutions but not the insurance arrangements, or insurance but not the institutions; or it may do neither, but merely provide a framework of rules and regulations within which health insurance and provider agencies operate.

In the organization of insurance-based health services, a distinction is commonly drawn between the 'direct' and 'indirect' pattern (Roemer 1969). In the direct pattern, an insurance agency provides health services in its own institutions, usually employing salaried medical personnel. This is the pattern that has developed in many Latin American countries. In the indirect pattern (prevalent in the United States and Europe but also in some developing countries), the insuring agency meets the cost of care given by private health care providers practising from facilities not owned by the insurer. Such an insurance system is referred to as a 'third party' payment system, since the insurance agency, as the 'third party', has no direct authority over the other two parties, the provider and the consumer. A variant of this pattern is possible, where the insurer contracts with publicly-provided facilities to care for the insured.

Social insurance has been expanded and adapted, especially in Western Europe, to the extent that the distinction between a 'national health insurance system' and a 'national health service system' is a narrow one. The payments by employees and employers can be considered not as insurance premiums but as an earmarked tax, and government contributions to the insurance fund are often sizeable. Indeed, if both systems provide care at no direct charge, their economic effect on consumer demand can be argued to be similar. However, national health insurance usually attempts to maintain a financially viable and actuarially sound system so that contributions are directly related to the cost of medical care. In addition, access to health care depends on the payment of contributions, whereas national health services usually have no eligibility rules (other than possibly registration with a general practitioner), and the only limit to access is the capacity of health facilities (Krizay and Wilson 1974). Finally, health insurance may finance certain benefits only (for instance hospital in-patient services) whereas a national health service commonly gives access to all publicly-provided services.

A major difference between the British national health service and the Western European health insurance-based systems stems from the integration of the financing and provider functions in Britain. However, if social insurance systems of the direct form, common in many developing countries, were eventually to be expanded to cover the great majority of the population, then they would become equivalent to national health service systems, though financed by an earmarked tax rather than general government revenues. It follows that the use of the term 'insurance' is to some extent misleading, since both systems of financing do provide insurance against the cost of health care. Ultimately, there-fore, the only distinction to be drawn between national health insurance, as conventionally financed through payroll taxes, and a national health service, is that they raise money by different methods. Yet this distinction is very important, for different ways of raising money have profound effects on the organization, efficiency, utilization, and equity of health care systems.

The economic implications of health insurance

The introduction of health insurance in either its private or social form into a developing country is likely to carry with it certain implications for the efficiency and equity of the health care system. This section attempts to analyse some of these implications, in order to reach an understanding on the likely behaviour of different institutional forms of health insurance.

This analysis necessarily demands exploration of whether health care possesses characteristics that distinguish it from goods and services normally produced and purchased in private markets, and whether health insurance has certain characteristics that distinguish it from other forms of insurance. The arguments relate essentially to *uncertainty* on the part of the individual on the type and quantity of health care needed; to the respective roles of *consumer* and *provider* in determining access to and consumption of health care; and to the role of *equity* considerations in influencing who should receive care and who should pay for it.

Uncertainty

The attraction of health insurance to an individual is that premiums are paid regularly in order that payments and potentially large financial losses should be avoided at the time of illness. But will the removal of direct payments lead individuals to demand more care than they would otherwise, for instance by indulging in more health-damaging activities, by visiting health facilities more frequently, or by consuming more care once they have decided to attend the clinic, pharmacy, or hospital?

These possibilities might appear implausible to those who consider that an individual's 'need' for health care is clear and unambiguous. Yet this notion makes economists uneasy unless it is stated clearly who determines need. Economists prefer in the first instance to talk not about need, but about demand, defined as the quantity of a commodity consumers wish and are able to buy at a given price (Lee 1979). This definition goes beyond the common notion of 'desire' or 'need', for unless desire is made effective by both *ability* and *willingness* to pay, it is not demand in the economic sense.

Demand for a product will be influenced by many variables, but one of the most important is likely to be its price. Assuming the other variables do not change, economic theory predicts that the higher the price, the smaller will be the quantity demanded of any product or service, and the lower the price, the larger the quantity demanded. This relationship can be expressed graphically, as in Fig. 4.1. The slope of the curve indicates how responsive is an individual's demand for a good to changes in its price. The extent to which demand changes in response to a change in price is termed by economists the 'elasticity of demand'. Assuming that consumers are rational, that is that they consistently

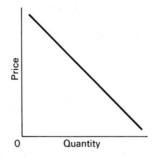

Fig. 4.1. An individual's demand curve for a good or service.

wish to maximize the total benefits they obtain from a given expenditure, consumers will compare the benefits of consuming one more unit of a good (its marginal value) with the cost or price of one more unit (its marginal cost). Given the financial resources at their command, they will expand consumption as long as marginal value exceeds marginal cost. Thus price is a major rationing mechanism upon demand.

This exposition (necessarily simplified) of the theory of demand can be built on to explore the likely behaviour of private markets for health care and to explore the impact of insurance on demand. In Fig. 4.2 the individual's demand for health care at different prices is shown by the curve DD[1] and the supply of health care by SS[1]. If the consumer faces a price for health care of P, and this is the only cost involved in obtaining care, he would consume up to the point where his marginal value equals the price, that is Q units. If, however, he faces no price, for instance because he is insured, he will increase his consumption to point D[1]. Yet at this point, his valuation of the extra units of health care is *less*

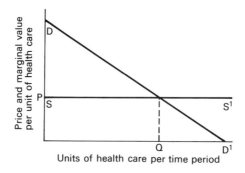

Fig. 4.2. An individual's demand for health care.

than the cost of producing them. In other words, his consumption is inefficiently high in his own value terms (though others may still place a higher value on his consumption).

How likely is this situation of 'over' consumption to exist in practice? The existence and magnitude of the change in demand when the consumer pays no direct price depends essentially on the shape of the demand curve, that is on the elasticity of demand. If the curve is vertical, as in Fig. 4.3, representing perfectly inelastic demand, the lowering of the price the consumer faces will have no impact on demand. If it slopes downwards, as in Fig. 4.2, it will increase the quantities demanded. The resolution of this issue, therefore, is a matter for empirical investigation. It is clear that price elasticities will vary between services (for instance between out-patient and in-patient services) and will be affected by the severity of the patient's condition. There is considerable literature, mainly American, devoted to these questions, and evidence that demand for health services is to some extent responsive to price changes (Kaplan and Lave 1971; Maynard 1979*a*).

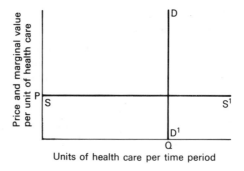

Fig. 4.3. An individual's perfectly inelastic demand for health care.

The above paragraphs have described what the insurance industry calls 'moral hazard'; that is the tendency of individuals, once insured, to behave in such a way as to increase the likelihood or size of the risk against which they have insured. From an individual's point of view such behaviour may be highly rational; indeed he may value insurance precisely because he does not wish to be faced with problems over ability or willingness to pay when he is ill (Brown 1981). However, from the insurer's point of view, such behaviour may lead to a larger quantity of care being consumed, and thus to higher costs which require higher premiums. In a developing country where only a small proportion of the population receive the benefits of health insurance, such a process can accentuate the already glaring differences that exist in the amount of health care received by different sections of the population.

There are well-developed methods used by the insurance industry to combat moral hazard. These include 'co-insurance', making the insured pay a proportion of his medical costs; 'deductibles', making the insured liable for the initial expenses up to a stated sum; and 'fixed indemnity', where an individual is insured for a given expenditure, usually for an illness or a year, but occasionally over his lifetime (Brandt, Horisberger, and von Wartburg 1980). Co-insurance is widely used in both developed and developing countries. In developing countries its purpose may be not only to limit demand, but also to make an insurance scheme financially viable when incomes are low. Considerable debate has taken place, especially in the United States, on the impact of cost-sharing upon health care utilization and on its efficiency and equity implications. There is evidence that the lower the cost-sharing rate, the larger will be demand; at the same time, there are fears that cost-sharing may deter those in 'need', and discourage early attendance, leading to more severe cases and greater expenditure on treatment later on (Mansinghka 1978; Maynard 1979*b*; Newhouse 1981). Deductibles, as an alternative to co-insurance, can be particularly useful to the insurer if applied to those services (such as drugs) which generate large volumes of small claims for reimbursement, and thus impose considerable administrative costs.

This analysis of the responsiveness of demand to price changes also suggests that the scope of insurance benefits covered can affect the composition as well as the level of demand. For example, if health insurance provides benefits for in-patient care only, demand will be biased away from out-patient care. Thus insurance, by changing the relative prices that consumers face for different health services, can either unintentionally distort the pattern of demand, or it can provide a positive opportunity to shape the demand in favour of cost-effective treatment patterns.

Finally, the impact of moral hazard in an insurance-financed system (or indeed a national health service) will depend not only on demand factors but also on the availability of supply and the response of providers. In a third-party payment system, an increase in demand is likely in the short run only to lead to a rise in prices, but in the long run to an increase in supply. If, however, providers can restrain the expansion of supply, and insuring agencies have limited influence on prices, the result may be cost inflation. Where insuring agencies can control the supply of services (as in the 'direct' pattern, or in 'prepayment' systems where a physician or hospital also acts as an insuring agency) moral hazard will be limited by supply restrictions and rationing, though at the risk of consumer dissatisfaction.

In conclusion, moral hazard has been considered a major problem in the context of developed countries, and fears of 'over-consumption' and cost inflation have prompted the development of mechanisms to ration available resources (WHO 1977). The problem of how to ration in the absence of price is even more acute in the developing world (witness complaints that free services lead to 'unnecessary' use) and the consequence of free services may be high demand that can swamp health facilities and increase costs. It is necessary, however, to explore further *who* is actually 'demanding' and *who* is actually determining utilization patterns.

Provider influence

Traditional economic theory assumes the substantial independence of demand and supply; in particular, that suppliers do not directly influence the quantity demanded. In the health sector, however, it is clear that doctors, as suppliers of medical care, do have considerable direct influence on consumption. In addition, it can be questioned whether or not consumers always have sufficient knowledge to judge whether they are in need of health care, and if so, what type and quantity of health care they require.

Some economists would argue that these points do not necessarily affect the consumer adversely in a private market for health care, if the doctor acts as the patient's agent and is influenced by him (Kaplan and Lowe 1971). However, the doctor's decisions are likely to reflect not only his patient's preferences but also his own, and particularly his preference for a reasonable income. In a private health care system or under any other forms of remuneration except direct salary, his income will be related to the nature and volume of services he supplies and to the price he receives for them (Evans 1974). A fee-for-service system, in particular, will provide strong incentives to an income-maximizing doctor to expand the quantity of services he provides, and to emphasize those which yield the highest fees. However, maximizing income is unlikely to be the only or the most important variable in what is termed the doctor's 'utility function'. Income, status, and leisure time are all likely to be significant (Lee and Mills 1982). Moreover, professional ethics and attitudes may be important in counteracting such incentives, and maintaining the status of the profession.

None the less, it is clear that doctors (and hospitals) do respond to the incentives inherent in different payment systems (Glaser 1970) and do constitute a significant influence on demand. It has been argued that the most realistic model of demand is where the consumer decides whether or not to enter the health system, and the doctor determines the treatment (Cullis and West 1979). In a private market, therefore, the lack of countervailing power by the consumer may permit overcharging and high-cost services, and/or the supply of an inefficiently large quantity of health care (i.e. over-consumption). The introduction of insurance cover would reduce the consumer's resistance both to seeking care and to receiving it. Where the provider is separate from the insurer (in the indirect system), insurance cover liberates the provider from having to tailor his treatment to the resources of the patient. That this is an important consideration is shown by the evidence of at least one developing country where doctors welcomed health insurance as a way of expanding their market (Seitz 1981), and this is probably true of others also.

This issue of the relative influence of providers and consumers has been discussed at some length because of its policy implications. If it is feared that the introduction of a health insurance system (or, indeed, a national health service), which reduces the cost of health care to the patient at the point of consumption, will lead to increased utilization and pressure on scarce health service resources, then the appropriate policy response may not be to introduce mechanisms to influence the consumer, but rather to consider ways of affecting the behaviour of providers. The institutional form of a health insurance system will therefore have a considerable impact on its efficiency.

Equity considerations

Equity is universally recognized as a major consideration affecting the organization and provision of health care, though the exact distribution of the financing burden and consumption of health care that constitutes 'equity' will vary from country to country. This section therefore concentrates on discussing the distributive consequences of health insurance, rather than on exploring the concept of equity *per se*.

In many societies it is assumed that consumers are the best judge of their own welfare, and should choose themselves which goods and services to consume. Thus it is considered more efficient to leave individuals to decide how to distribute their own income than to insist they purchase a particular good that they may not want. However, there are well established circumstances under which societies recognize departures from these rules. In particular, consumers make choices on the basis of a given distribution of income and wealth. While society may not care how much meat is consumed once basic nutritional requirements are met, or how many pencils are purchased, there are good grounds for assuming that societies do care whether individuals receive health care when ill, and whether the health care provided is adequate.

It is likely that if individuals were left to purchase the health care they want with the income available to them, some would be unable to afford what would be considered, in the context of any particular country, an appropriate amount. Moreover, the purchasing power of poor communities may be inadequate to attract health practitioners and facilities, as has been reported, for instance, for Korea (Park and Yeon 1981). The problem comes in determining how to move towards a different distribution of health care consumption than that which results from 'free' market forces. Furthermore, once income transfers are made to subsidize consumption, attention has to be given not only to who is *consuming* health care but also to who is *paying*.

In the circumstances described above, private health insurance is unlikely to be a solution. Private insurance agencies will relate premiums to the actuarial risk of the individual. If they do not, they will be subsidizing high-risk individuals by 'over-charging' low risks. The latter may then be attracted away by agencies offering lower premiums, unless community rating is enforced on all insuring agencies (forcing low-risk individuals to subsidize high risks). Thus private insurance is highly unlikely to cover bad risks such as those with chronic diseases, the elderly, and, indeed, low-income groups who usually have worse health than the better off. In most developed countries, and even in the United States where private insurance is widespread, social insurance is provided for such groups. The alternative, of enabling low-income groups and high risks to insure themselves, for instance, through income supplements or vouchers for purchasing health insurance, is notoriously difficult to implement in practice, even in developed countries.

The organization of health insurance on a public, that is governmental basis, however, does not necessarily ensure an equitable system, and in countries where social insurance schemes exist, there are a number of ways in which their operation has been condemned as inequitable. Even if social insurance covers both high and low wage earners, utilization patterns will not necessarily be proportional to health need. Paying a price for health care can be viewed as a rationing device; when care is free at the point of consumption, rationing by waiting and by the providers of care will replace rationing by price. The equity of the system will depend firstly on how different income groups value the cost of waiting: for instance, is it less for lower-income groups because the opportunity cost of their time is less; or is it less for higher paid workers because they are paid a salary not an hourly wage? Secondly, it will depend on whom the providers select or attract for treatment. Evidence from Britain shows that despite the availability of 'free' care, low-income groups, in relation to their health need, consume less than their fair share of health services (Black 1980).

Differential utilization patterns need to be matched with the distribution of the financing burden within the insurance scheme to assess total internal redistribution effects. Taxes can be regressive (they take a decreasing proportion of income as income rises), progressive (they take an increasing proportion of income as income rises), or proportional (they take a constant proportion at all income levels). If the payroll taxes used conventionally to finance social insurance are flat-rate (that is a constant amount regardless of income) then their effect will be highly regressive. Even if they are a constant percentage of income they are likely to be regressive because there is usually a maximum contribution; the contribution is levied only on wages and salaries and not on other forms of income; and any co-payment arrangements for care are likely to represent a higher proportion of the income of the poor than of the rich (Bodenheimer 1973). Since payroll taxes represent a system of payment that is not directly related to health risk, their redistributive effects are quite different from those of private insurance based on the actuarial risk of the individual; payroll taxes are likely to produce a much greater redistribution from the healthy to the sick than a private scheme.

Other redistributive effects can result from the distribution of the financing burden of social insurance amongst the population at large. For instance, while it is commonly assumed that the employee contribution to the payroll tax falls on the worker and is not transferred, the employer contribution may be shifted to the workers through lower wages, or to consumers through raising the prices of goods sold. If the latter, then the incidence of the tax depends on the income levels of those who purchase the goods and on their willingness to continue to purchase them. Moreover many governments subsidize insurance from general tax revenues or by giving tax concessions on insurance premiums. A social insurance scheme that covers only a small proportion of the population may therefore turn out to be financed partly by those outside the scheme who purchase goods whose prices are higher, and partly by those who pay government taxes.

In defence, it has been argued that social insurance represents a net addition to a country's health care resources, and by example helps to raise the standards of health care for those outside the schemes, especially the urban and rural poor (Roemer and Maeda 1976). None the less, the purchasing power harnessed by social insurance may attract skilled manpower in short supply (such as doctors and nurses) to cater for those who might otherwise be most vocal in pressing for improvements in public health services.

Finally, it is important to keep in mind the efficiency consequences of any taxation arrangements that are designed to promote an equitable social insurance system. Any tax will have an effect on the economic behaviour of the taxpayer. In developing countries, there is a danger that payroll taxes, by increasing the cost of labour and often the relative cost of low wage-earners, may lead the employer to substitute capital inputs for labour, and highly skilled for low skilled workers. On the other hand, in economies short of skilled labour, social insurance may be seen as providing important and necessary 'fringe' benefits which help to attract skilled and professional workers.

Institutional forms of health insurance: the United States

Before considering the ways in which not-for-profit health insurance and social insurance can be, and are, organized in developing countries, some useful lessons can be drawn about insurance-based health care systems by looking at experiences in the United States. A major feature of the health system in the United States is its complexity. Over 90 per cent of Americans have some form of health insurance, provided either privately (largely by non-profit agencies) or by government assistance through Medicaid (for the poor) and Medicare (for the elderly). With some exceptions (discussed later), insurance agencies are separate from provider agencies.

One of the most publicized features of the United States health care system over the last two decades or so, and of great concern at present within the United States, has been its rates of cost inflation (Hurst 1982). Between 1965 and 1978, per capita expenditure on health rose by 397 per cent and on hospitals by 484 per cent (Intriligator 1981), which in aggregate terms has meant that by the late 1970s nearly 10 per cent of GNP was devoted to health. These increases have been ascribed more to price than quantity changes. While there is considerable argument over the causative influences producing this cost inflation, it is generally agreed that it was at the very least made possible because the paying agencies (third-party insurers and governments) merely reimbursed the costs of hospitals. Behind this fact lie a number of influences. Increased private and public insurance cover (especially resulting from the government programmes of Medicare and Medicaid and from tax subsidies for private insurance cover) raised patient demand for health care. Hospitals responded to this changing situation by increasing capacity, a further stimulus to demand, and physicians, paid on a fee-for-service basis and knowing their patients were insured, also faced incentives to treat more patients and provide more services per patient. At the same time, the medical profession remained restricted in numbers by barriers to entry including control of numbers in training and the length of training. As a result, unit costs rose.

Neither consumers, providers, nor insurers appeared to feel the need to restrain these costs. Most consumers of private insurance received cover as a fringe benefit from employment and many were in non-contributory schemes, that is the full cost of insurance was met by their employers who did not exert much pressure against premium increases (Sapolsky, Altman, Greene, and Moore 1981). Moreover, there was often extensive low-risk coverage, increasing further the potential demand for health services and leading to high administrative costs for insurance companies. In addition, the link between increased utilization and rising premiums was unclear for any particular consumer (even if he paid part of the premium), and since most hospitalization insurance had no co-payment clauses, consumers had no incentive to shop around for good-value insurance packages, to economize on care, or to seek the more efficient and thus least-cost hospitals (Newhouse 1981).

Up to the 1970s, providers therefore faced no resistance to increasing supply and apparently few constraints on the prices they could charge. In particular, insurers and the government were disinclined or ill-equipped to challenge the dominant position of the medical profession, and faced little consumer, trade union, or employer resistance to rising premiums. More recently, Federal and State Governments have attempted to control costs through the regulation of prices or the quantity of services provided, with varying degrees of success (Feldstein 1979; Hurst 1982). Cost containment still remains a major source of concern:

Existing financial and reimbursement arrangements provide incentives for the public to seek and providers to deliver more care than knowledgeable physicians deem appropriate or necessary; for hospitals to be overbuilt; for technology to run rampant; and for costs, prices and expenditure to keep escalating (Fein 1980).

While there appears to be general agreement that a major problem exists, opinions vary on whether more effective cost containment will be achieved by greater competition free of government involvement, or by a stronger regulatory role for government.

There are a number of important lessons that developing countries can learn from this experience. First, insurance, by lowering the cost of care at the point of delivery, is likely to increase demand for both a greater quantity of health services and for higher quality services. Secondly, there will be a correlation between the use of deductibles or co-insurance and reduced hospitalization, though the greater the influence of providers, the weaker this correlation is likely to be. Thirdly, if the insuring agency has little control over the number of services used and their cost, the introduction or expansion of health insurance can lead to an appreciable rise in costs. Fourthly, when insurance cover is not comprehensive, for instance favouring hospital in-patient rather than out-patient care, it will bias treatment towards insured services. Finally, experience in the United States demonstrates the complexity of the determinants underlying the demand and supply of medical care, and the difficulties public agencies can face if they attempt to either regulate or encourage competitive behaviour in a market with strong vested interests.

Any attempt to relate American experience to developing countries must clearly take account of the differences in their levels of health and health care expenditure. While increased utilization may be considered questionable in a country such as the United States where levels of health and provision are already high, the improvement of levels of provision is often a national policy in a developing country. However, where the insurance sector treats only a selected minority of the population and provides an increased quantity and quality of care for the insured, with correspondingly higher unit costs, then such costs can make it extremely difficult to expand insurance coverage or to extend public health services to cater for the majority of the population (Zschock 1982).

Mounting criticism of the various institutional forms of health insurance in the United States has stimulated a search for innovative forms which are compatible with a decentralized, pluralist health system but which provide incentives for cost containment and efficiency. One such innovation is the prepayment system, where the insuring agency and provider are the same institution (Krizay and Wilson 1974). The consumer pays an annual subscription (that is, an insurance premium) and in return is offered comprehensive care. The providing agency has a financial incentive to limit 'unnecessary' care; indeed, studies have suggested that prepaid group practices can be more cost-effective than fee-for-service systems, largely because of lower hospitalization rates (Saward and Fleming 1980). Since such practices demand considerable capital investment and a large catchment population, health maintenance organizations (HMOs) have been developed as an alternative system; a primary care doctor provides all primary care services, purchases and supervises all other health care, and in return receives a capitation payment from each consumer (Enthoven 1980; Luft 1981). Yet, despite the considerable praise they have received from policy makers and academics, HMOs have enrolled only about 4 per cent of the United States population.

Though prepayment systems and HMOs have had only limited success, two points are worthy of special note. First, the integration of the insurance and provider functions corresponds closely to the 'direct' pattern of health insurance in developing countries. While a major stimulus for the direct pattern is likely to have been the lack of alternative facilities for the insured population, this point of similarity underlines the potential advantage the direct pattern enjoys in cost containment. However, the incentive for cost containment in HMOs has two major sources: the amalgamation of the insurer and provider functions, and competition for subscribers with other HMOs and conventional insurance agencies. The latter aspect is not a common feature of the direct system, which usually possesses a captive population.

Secondly, the adoption of a capitation fee divorces the doctor's clinical management of a patient from his form of remuneration. The advantages of such a separation have been recognized for some time. In India, for example, the employment of salaried doctors to treat insured patients was advocated in 1944, and subsequently implemented wherever feasible (Singh 1982). Where this was not possible, a panel doctor was paid on a capitation, not fee-for-service, basis. Such systems of payment carry, of course, their own potential dangers: for capitation payments, that of maximizing the number of people registered and minimizing the services they receive; and for salaries, of minimizing activities. The question is whether or not such disincentives are to be preferred to a system which encourages providers to maximize the number of services they provide. Any country will necessarily have to work out its own system of payment in the light of these and other factors that influence the behaviour of providers.

Health insurance in developing countries

This final section of the chapter concentrates on three factors that are of particular importance when analysing insurance systems: coverage of the population; health care coverage; and institutional structures. Particular attention is also given to innovative forms of health insurance that might tackle the equity and efficiency shortcomings of many existing systems.

Coverage of the population

Social insurance schemes are concentrated in the industrial sector of developing countries not least because wages and profits are high enough for compulsory levies to be paid, and the structure of wage employment makes collection of the levies feasible. That sector, however, typically employs only a small proportion of the country's labour force, though in addition government workers may also be covered by insurance arrangements paid for by the government from its tax revenues, sometimes assisted by employee contributions. In Columbia, for example, the two insurance systems for private and public sector employees account for 50 per cent of health sector expenditure, yet cover at most 25 per cent of the population (Zschock 1979). A similar pattern is evident in other Latin American countries: while figures on health sector finance are generally very scanty (see Chapter 3), it is clear that social insurance systems control a large part of health service resources, some of which are paid in the form of government subsidies, while providing care to a small proportion of the total population.

The extension of social insurance to rural or peri-urban areas faces many problems. The majority of working populations in developing countries are either self-employed or work for small enterprises in the agricultural, petty trade, artisan, and service sectors. In the urban informal sector, wages are typically low and employment unstructured. In the agricultural sector also, incomes are often low, may be received in kind rather than cash and may be spread over a larger number of economically inactive household members than in urban areas. When, as is often the case, small-scale agricultural or industrial producers face prices set by the market which they cannot influence, they may be unable to pass on the cost of insurance to consumers, and any payroll tax may threaten their financial viability. Moreover, the per capita cost of health care in rural areas is likely to be higher than in urban areas, requiring larger payments for the same level of services, and an administrative structure that can be used for the collection of contributions may not exist.

There are, however, a number of ways in which either compulsory or voluntary insurance schemes could be set up to include rural populations (though not usually the informal urban sector). These schemes are usually dependent on breaking the link between insurance and payroll taxes. For instance, the contributions of self-employed farmers can be linked to the size of farm and type of crop (thus avoiding the problem of determining income directly); low-interest loans can be given to assist the payment of contributions in those months when incomes are low; or if crops are marketed by a co-operative, or a co-operative bank provides credit, these organizations can be used to collect contributions when the harvest is marketed or credit repaid (Mallett 1980). In Mexico, agricultural credit societies pay annual contributions for all their members (Savy 1978), and in Japan, a rural health insurance scheme is financed through local household taxation and state subsidies (Higuchi 1974). Of particular value, since they simplify collection mechanisms, are taxes that are levied on communal or co-operative sources of income. For instance in Brazil, a tax on the value of agricultural products sold (that is, an earmarked tax) is paid to local hospitals which in return admit rural workers and their dependants as 'insured persons' (Bastos 1971; Roemer 1973).

The financial viability of such schemes depends on the balance between income and expenditure. Only in very prosperous areas are farmers likely to be able to afford payments that can finance both primary and secondary care. Two solutions are commonly proposed: the first is to rely on state subsidies to supplement household contributions and to make up for the absence of employers' contributions; the second is to require cost-sharing, especially for secondary care. Cost-sharing is frequently expected in conventional social insurance schemes, for instance in the Philippines and Korea, but can be employed also in rural schemes, as in China.

Indeed, the example of China is worth exploring at some length, since it displays a number of features relevant to expanded coverage and has been described in detail by Hu (1981). The insurance covering rural communes, entitled 'co-operative medical services', is said to cover 70 per cent of communes. Once a commune has decided to join the scheme, membership of commune members is compulsory. Premiums paid by family members amount to on average 1.5 per cent of family disposable income, and contributions are also paid from collective funds. A small fee is charged for each visit to the brigade health station, and if a patient is referred to a county or city hospital by a barefoot doctor, part of the hospital fee (for instance 50 per cent or a fixed sum) will be reimbursed by the brigade health fund, and a low-interest loan may be provided to assist with payment of the balance (Wen and Hays 1976). Financial assistance is also provided by production team funds (for the salaries of barefoot doctors and public health workers) and by state funds (mainly for capital expenditure on local hospitals and clinics).

While conclusions on the success of such a system must be tentative in view of the lack of information on its actual operation, the Chinese system of rural insurance does suggest that such arrangements can be financially feasible if contributions are collected from a number of sources including government sources for hospitals, if substantial cost-sharing is expected for secondary care, and if low-cost forms of care are provided. As a guide to what families might be able and willing to pay in poor communities, it is interesting to note that for water supply projects, one loan agency has come to the conclusion that families are rarely able to pay more than 5 per cent of their income for water charges (World Bank 1976).

Health care coverage

An alternative approach to tailoring insurance schemes to suit resource availability is to limit the scope of benefits. The possibility of using the insurance principle to finance primary health care has appeared attractive to both national governments and international agencies, who are becoming increasingly aware that achieving 100 per cent coverage for primary health care demands substantial resources (Cumper 1980). Traditional medical care, the only form of care at present available to many rural communities, is usually paid for on a fee-for-service basis, suggesting that commuting such payments at least partially into health insurance may be feasible, where efficient organizations can be set up to handle the finance. The proceedings of a WHO/UNICEF conference on the cost of primary health care (WHO/UNICEF 1980) indicate that a number of countries are experimenting with community-based insurance systems. Their success is likely to depend to a considerable extent on the existence of strong local organizations, as in China, in the form of workers' councils, co-operatives, or farmers' unions, to control, organize and manage the insurance system.

It is apparent that if premiums are low enough for the majority of the population to afford them, and if the services provided are geared to the income from premiums, not-for-profit insurance can be used to develop local services controlled by local organizations. However, while adopting a scheme may be voluntary, it is likely that, as in China, membership of a local scheme may need to be compulsory, in order that the burden of risk be spread, and that low-risk or high-income individuals should not opt out. The problems will arise in the financing of more sophisticated services, where government support is likely to be needed.

In contrast to rural areas, where low incomes are likely to limit the range of care that can be financed by insurance, urban-based social insurance schemes have been widely criticized for concentrating largely on curative, in-patient care, and neglecting less costly forms of curative care and preventive care. Clearly this is always likely to be the outcome where those insured insist upon sophisticated services, when insurance agencies have little control over the quantity of services provided, and when facilities are provided indirectly and can thus respond to this demand. A curative, high-cost pattern of service can also result from insurance cover which is limited to the more expensive (usually hospital) services.

Institutional structures

Some of the relative merits of indirect and direct systems of insurance have already been identified. From the economist's perspective, what is important is to determine which system is most likely to produce health care efficiently. Roemer has argued strongly that not only does the direct pattern produce better quality care, but also that it does so more efficiently, particularly in its use of paramedical and auxiliary staff (Roemer 1969). Moreover, the direct pattern avoids the problem faced by third-party insurers of attempting to find a method of payment for doctors and hospitals that promotes efficient behaviour. Whilst the salaries and hospital budgets usually favoured by the direct pattern are not ideal, particularly since salaries may not provide a sufficient incentive for high productivity, they do at least facilitate cost control. In contrast, reimbursement methods such as fee-for-service and fees per patient day do not encourage physicians or hospital managers to ration the quantity of services given to patients. In Brazil, for example, a recent study has shown that much of the variation in Caesarian section rates in the maternity units of a number of hospitals can be associated with the financial status of the patient: rates were 75 per cent of deliveries for private patients, 40 per cent of deliveries for insured patients, and less than 25 per cent for indigent patients (Janowitz, Nakamura, Lins, Brown, and Clopton 1982).

While the merits of the direct pattern have frequently been emphasized, it is not without defects. It is often organized as a separate enclave, quite distinct institutionally from the health care services of other agencies, especially of the Ministry of Health. For instance in Latin America, in 15 out of 20 schemes, responsibility for administrative supervision lay with the Ministry of Labour or of Social Welfare and in another three, while the Ministry of Health exercized general supervision, services were directly administered by social security institutions (Roemer 1973). Furthermore, many countries have multiple insurance systems, each system with its own services and catering for different groups of workers or even different government departments. Such structures tend to create access problems for those eligible for services and encourage the duplication of facilities. They may also have high administrative costs since each scheme is relatively small and is therefore unable to take advantage of economies of scale that can be enjoyed by large insurance agencies.

The co-ordination or unification of separate insurance funds and the linkage of insurance schemes to the Ministry of Health is therefore now recommended (WHO 1971). Integration of health services for the insured with public health services can be achieved by insisting, for instance, that social insurance agencies should provide medical and allied services partly or wholly through existing facilities and personnel of the Ministry of Health, strengthening these with subsidies for capital and recurrent expenditure. Thus in Jordan, civil servants receive care in public hospitals without charge, in return for a monthly salary deduction paid to the Ministry of Health. This type of system is clearly quite difficult to set up when Ministry of Health services are inadequate, though even so capital funds could be devoted to expanding existing services rather than setting up separate facilities for the insured. Yet the problem may remain that insured people expect, by virtue of their payment contribution, to receive a better standard of care than that available in Ministry of Health facilities. An important issue is whether their demands can be partially met by providing improved ward accommodation and fringe benefits but without the provision of separate treatment and diagnostic facilities.

While it is possible to generalize about the advantages of these three patterns of organization, the indirect, the direct, and the joint Ministry of Health/health insurance system, a country's choice of health insurance scheme will clearly depend on the existing pattern of services, their ownership and payment systems. Two major considerations are likely to be the presence or absence of a substantial private medical system, and the adequacy of public health services. The possibilities open to countries with a different inheritance can be explored by taking the examples of Korea and Tunisia.

In Korea, most physicians work on a private, fee-for-service basis, and the majority of hospital beds are privately owned and concentrated in urban areas (Park and Yeon 1981). Over 85 per cent of health expenditure is financed by consumers, and until 1977, when a medical insurance programme was set up, Korea had no financial mechanisms for pooling risks (apart from a few pilot programmes). By 1981, the medical insurance programme required firms with at least a hundred workers, government officials, teachers, and ancillary staff of private schools, to be compulsorily insured and provided for a voluntary, community-based programme for all others. Within four years, 28 per cent of the population have been covered by insurance. The private pattern of health services has been retained, providers being remunerated according to a specified fee schedule. However, the insurance system has:

begun to redirect private expenditure into what promises to be a less costly and more equitable system of health care than direct payments for private medicine (Zschock 1982).

In Tunisia, it appears that reasonable public facilities were available when medical care coverage under social security was introduced. It was therefore possible to arrange that in return for an annual subsidy paid to the Ministry of Health by the social security agency, care would be provided through the regular public hospitals and health services. Insured workers were not to receive preferential treatment, but were exempt from fees normally charged (WHO 1971).

Summary and conclusion

Two main themes have been running through this chapter: the advantages and disadvantages of insurance mechanisms for financing health care; and the relative merits of the involvement of public as against private institutions in health care. The experiences of insurance in the developed and developing world have been rather different. Western European health insurance, organized by public organizations or not-for-profit funds, has gradually expanded to near 100 per cent coverage of the population, and finances the purchase of health care from largely private agencies. Only a few European countries have abandoned insurance in favour of funding from general tax revenues, public ownership of facilities, and salaried employees. In the United States, social insurance is confined to the poor and elderly, private insurance agencies cater for a large proportion of the population, and health facilities are largely provided via the private market. Developing countries display many different patterns of organization and health care provision in their social security schemes covering medical care. In many, governments have taken a direct role in the financing and provision of a limited network of public health facilities, and insurance has been used as the means to expand health care for regular wage earners in the public and private sectors, either by enabling them to obtain care from independent or public providers, or by the direct provision of health care services. Most recently, interest has grown in insurance as a way of financing primary health care largely, though not necessarily exclusively, in rural areas.

Whether private or public systems of health care are likely to work more efficiently can be considered as much an ideological issue as one susceptible to empirical assessment. There is increasing agreement amongst economists, however, that whatever the structure of health care, it is likely to be as important to concentrate on encouraging efficiency and cost effectiveness in provider agencies as to rely upon influencing consumer behaviour through measures such as cost sharing. Two important questions for developing countries, therefore, are firstly, what organizational pattern provides the right incentives to doctors and other health personnel to be cost effective and to look for ways of delivering better care at less cost; and secondly which pattern meets, or does not contradict, the equity objectives of countries.

The value of insurance as a principle, providing protection for the individual against the cost of illness, is clear. Beyond that principle, the value of an insurance system depends on its effect both as a source of funds and as a way of organizing the provision of health care. Its effect can be evaluated in terms of:

(1) the distribution of the financing burden (costs) over the population, and the extent to which insurance facilitates access to, and utilization of, health services (benefits) by different groups in the population;
(2) the quantity and quality of the services it finances, and the feasibility of extending coverage of such services to the whole population within a reasonable time period;
(3) the efficiency of these services, that is the provision of care at least cost;
(4) the efficiency of health insurance administration; and
(5) the extent to which health insurance assists the achievement of national policy objectives.

This chapter has noted that health insurance, both private and public, direct and indirect, has been condemned on many of these counts in international circles. Such shortcomings have prompted much advice on what the appropriate circumstances might be for health care coverage to be safely introduced or expanded through a form of social security (Roemer 1971; WHO 1971, 1978; Zschock 1982). In the meantime, many governments of developing countries still look to health insurance, if only as a way of supplementing public revenues for health care, or of harnessing direct consumer payments.

Insurance clearly can be used, and indeed is used, as a way of providing services to those in the modern sector of the economy. So long as the distributive effect of such care does not violate notions of equity, and the health services for the insured do not detract from the care available for other sections of the population, then social insurance can be instrumental in raising resources for the health sector and enabling certain groups to finance their health care needs themselves. Social insurance can also be used to ensure either that these resources are not channelled into a private health sector, whose growth could cause even greater inequity and inefficiency if consumers are uninformed and providers unconstrained, or that the use made of an existing private sector, and its behaviour, is directed towards meeting national objectives. Finally, the limited ability of many governments to increase taxation, and the often low priority given to health expenditure in rural areas and for the urban poor, provide strong reasons for looking closely at the possibility of using voluntary insurance to develop local level, and in particular, primary health services.

REFERENCES

Abel-Smith, B. (1978). Poverty, development and health policy. *Publ. Hlth Pap. WHO* **69**.
— (1981). Health care in a cold economic climate. *Lancet* 373–6.
Bastos, M. V. (1971). Brazil's multiple social insurance programs and their influence on medical care. *Int. J. Hlth Serv.* **1**, 378–89.
Black, D. (1980). *Inequalities in health: report of a research working group.* Department of Health and Social Security, London.
Blanpain, J. (1978). *National health insurance and health resources.* Harvard University Press.
Bodenheimer, T. S. (1973). Health care in the US: who pays? *Int. J. Hlth Serv.* **3**, 427–34.
Brandt, A., Horisberger, B., and von Wartburg, W. P. (1980). *Cost-sharing in health care.* Springer-Verlag, Berlin.
Brown, L. D. (1981). Competition and health cost containment: cautions and conjectures. *Milbank Meml Fund Q. Bull.* (Health and Society), **59**, 145–89.
Culyer, A. J. (1972). The 'market' versus the 'state' in medical care. In *Problems and progress in medical care*, 7 (ed. G. McLachlan). Oxford University Press.
— (1976). *Need and the national health service.* Martin Robertson, London.
Cullis, J. G. and West, P. A. (1979). *The economics of health.* Martin Robertson, London.
Cumper, G. (1980). *Primary health care and the resources for health development.* Background Paper for Joint WHO/UNICEF Interregional Conference on the Costs of Primary Health Care, Geneva, 1980.
Enthoven, A. C. (1980). Health care cost control through incentives and competition. In *Cost-sharing in health care* (ed. A. Brandt, B. Horisberger, and W. P. von Wartburg). Springer-Verlag, Berlin.
Evans, R. G. (1974). Supplier-induced demand: some empirical evidence and implications. In *The economics of health and medical care* (ed. M. Perlman). Macmillan, London.
Fein, R. (1980). Social and economic attitudes shaping American health policy. *Milbank Meml Fund Q. Bull.* (Health and Society) **58**, 349–85.
Feldstein, P. J. (1979). *Health care economics.* Wiley, Chichester.
Glaser, W. A. (1970). *Paying the doctor: systems of remuneration and their effects.* Johns Hopkins Press, Baltimore.
Higuchi, T. (1974). Medical care through social insurance in the Japanese rural sector. *Int. Labour Rev.* **109**, 251–74.

Hu, T. -W. (1981). Issues of health care financing in the People's Republic of China. *Soc. Sci. Med.* **15C**, 233-7.

Hurst, J. W. (1982) An introduction to the American health care financing debate. Paper presented to the UK Health Economists Study Group, Brunel, July.

Intriligator, M. D. (1981). Major policy issues in the economics of health care in the United States. In *Health, economics and health economics* (ed. J. van der Gaag and M. Perlman). North-Holland, Amsterdam.

Janowitz, B., Nakamura, M. S., Lins, F. E., Brown, M. L., and Clopton, D. (1982). Caesarian section in Brazil. *Soc. Sci. Med.* **16**, 19-25.

Kaplan, R. S. and Lave, L. B. (1971). Patient incentives and hospital insurance. *Hlth Serv. Res.* **6**, 288-300.

Kohn, R. (1980). Strategies for change: finance and regulation. In *Economics and health policy* (ed. A. Griffiths and Z. Bankowski). The Council for International Organizations of Medical Sciences (CIOMS) and Sandoz Institute, Geneva.

Krizay, J. and Wilson, A. (1974). *The patient as consumer: health care financing in the U.S.* Lexington Books, D. C. Heath and Company, Lexington, Mass.

Lee, K. (1979). Need versus demand: the planner's dilemma. In *Economics and health planning* (ed. K. Lee). Croom Helm, London.

— and Mills, A. (1982). *Policy-making and planning in the health sector.* Croom Helm, London.

Luft, H. S. (1981). *Health maintenance organisations: dimensions of performance.* Wiley, New York.

Mallett, A. (1980). Social protection of the rural population. *Int. Soc. Security Rev.* **XXIII** (3/4), 359-93.

Mansinghka, S. K. (1978). *National health insurance issues: viability of cost-sharing concept.* Roche Laboratories, New York.

Maynard, A. (1979*a*). Pricing, demanders and the supply of health care. *Int. J. Hlth Serv.* **9**, 121-33.

— (1979*b*). Pricing, insurance and the national health service. *J. social Policy* **8**, 157-76.

Newhouse, J. P. (1981). The demand for medical care services: a retrospect and prospect. In *Health, economics and health economics* (ed. J. van der Gaag and M. Perlman). North-Holland, Amsterdam.

Park, C. K. and Yeon, H. S. (1981). Recent developments in the health care system of Korea. *Int. Soc. Security Rev.* **XXXIV(2/81)**, 151-67.

Roemer, M. I. (1969). *The organisation of medical care under social security.* International Labour Organization, Geneva.

— (1971). Social security for medical care: is it justified in developing countries? *Int. J. Hlth Serv.* **1**, 354-61.

— (1973). Development of medical services under social security in Latin America. *Int. Labour Rev.* **108**, 1-23.

— and Maeda, N. (1976). Does social security support for medical care weaken public health programmes? *Int. J. Hlth Serv.* **6**, 69-78.

Sapolsky, H. M., Altman, D., Greene, R., and Moore, J. D. (1981). Corporate attitudes towards health care costs. *Milbank Meml Fund Q. Bull.* (Health and Society) **59**, 561-85.

Savy, R. (1978). *Social security in agriculture.* International Labour Organization, Geneva.

Saward, E. W. and Fleming, S. (1980). Health maintenance organisations. *Scient. Am.* **243**, 37-43.

Scotton, R. B. (1974). *Medical care in Australia*. Sun Books, Melbourne.

Seitz, R. H. (1981). Health insurance in the Philippines. *Far East Health*, June.

Singh, H. M. (1982). Methods of medical care delivery: the experience of India. *Int. Soc. Security Rev.* **XXXV(1/82)**, 17-37.

Torrens, P. R. (1982). Some potential hazards of unplanned expansion of private health insurance in Britain. *Lancet* 29-31.

Wen, C. -P. and Hays, C. W. (1976). Health care financing in China. *Medical Care* **XIV(3)**, 241-54.

WHO (World Health Organization) (1971). Personal health care and social security. *Tech. Rep. Ser. Wld Hlth Org.* **480**.

— (1977). Containing the rising cost of medical care under social security. *WHO Chron.* **31**, 408-12.

— (1978). Financing of health services. *Tech. Rep. Ser. Wld Hlth Org.* **625**.

— /UNICEF (1980). *Report of interregional workshop on cost and financing patterns of primary health care*. World Health Organization, Geneva.

World Bank (1976). *Village water supply: a world bank paper*, World Bank, Washington DC.

Zschock, D. K. (1979). *Health care financing in developing countries*. APHA Monograph No. 1.

— (1982). General review of problems of medical care delivery under social security in developing countries. *Int. Soc. Security Rev.* **XXXV(1/82)**, 3-15.

Author's note

The author is indebted to the Jordanian Government and to the Overseas Development Administration, United Kingdom, for an opportunity to study health insurance systems at first hand in Jordan, and for providing the impetus for further work.

5

Resources and costs in primary health care

Kenneth Lee

Introduction

In modern times, health services have shown themselves only too capable of absorbing an increasing share of the resources that nations, both developed and developing, have created for public and private investment and consumption. Historically, in the developed world, it has proved possible to finance such resources from economic growth; indeed, the scale of health care expenditure in the developed world has been permitted, in large part, only by its economic prosperity. In many developing countries, however, rather different concerns arise from the ever-present context of tight financial constraints, and from their attempts to meet demands for the extension of primary health care to their entire populations at a cost both governments and populations can afford.

World-wide attention and debate is now being directed to the role of primary health care in society. The major theme of such attention has largely been the great health needs of the developing countries and the inappropriateness of a desire for, and the provision of, sophisticated medical technologies and institutions concentrated in urban settings. Indeed, there has been a growing disenchantment with the part that medical science has played, and can play, in improving people's health, and a demand that greater emphasis be placed upon, say, improving nutrition, or better environmental conditions. The virtue of the primary health care approach, at least as seen by its advocates, is that it consciously places greater emphasis upon health-improving (rather than disease-reducing) activities than do high technology models, and upon health rather than medical services in the drive to reduce morbidity and mortality (Lee and Mills 1982).

High levels of morbidity and mortality are, of course, much influenced by the political structure and complexion of a country. Hence, the concept of primary health care depends at least partly for its success upon being acceptable to those having the power to bring about its implementation. What is clear, therefore, is that developing countries do have a political choice between either strengthening their existing (often medical care) delivery systems or reorientating them in the light of known health needs and perceived levels of effectiveness towards a primary health care approach.

At the same time, there is considerable ambiguity surrounding the term 'primary health care'. Indeed, primary health care connotes different things to different people in different countries, and even in the same country. Conceptually, some argue that activities such as anti-poverty measures, food production and distribution, water, sanitation, housing, environmental protection, and education all contribute to health and, hence, should be seen as an integral part of the primary health care network. Others would wish to draw the boundaries of primary health care more tightly, if only to make its planning and implementation more attainable and manageable. Hence, the basic issue is to determine the aims and objectives of such health care, its scope and role, and its *modus operandi*.

Not surprisingly, developing countries have not always chosen the same strategies for the provision of primary health care. In the first place, they exhibit different methods and sources of financing primary health care, different patterns of delivering primary health care, and different mechanisms for remunerating primary health care workers. The merits and de-merits of some of these strategies, in terms of cost and resources, are considered in this chapter. In the second place, developing countries exhibit different organizational systems and, within them, different configurations of primary health care. Some systems actively encourage access, others have introduced barriers to access so their patterns of coverage, utilization, and systems of rationing will differ. Thirdly, and above all, political systems affect the degree to which there has been, and can be, changes in existing primary health care systems (Sidel and Sidel 1977). Again, some of these factors are considered in this chapter.

There does appear to be a common international commitment to the concept of primary health care, yet the variety of organizational structures and staffing patterns observed in developing countries defies any attempts to search and find the universal 'right answer'. Organizational structures and manning levels do differ considerably between, and within, developing countries. Hence, alternative strategies (such as choice of appropriate technologies, possible role re-allocations) should be discussed and decided upon in terms both of their resource and cost implications and their likely benefits. This chapter aims to add to that debate by addressing itself to a number of key economic issues that have emerged or are likely to arise in the developing world, in securing resources for, and meeting the costs of, primary health care.

Primary health care initiatives

Major differences exist between developing countries in terms of their political philosophy, socioeconomic development, history, natural resources, and geography, all of which will shape and influence the finance, structure, and processes of health care delivery. At the same time, it can be posited that, despite these very real differences, the problems and issues of primary health care are similar and so are the broad strategies for their solution. If there is any substance in that viewpoint, then it may not be necessary to distinguish too closely between developing countries in analysing primary health care issues.

That belief seemingly underpinned the Declaration of Alma Ata adopted by an International Conference on Primary Health Care, jointly sponsored and organized by WHO and UNICEF (WHO 1978*a*). This Declaration called on all governments to formulate national policies, strategies, and plans of action to launch and sustain primary health care as an integral part of a comprehensive national health system. Indeed, primary health care was seen as the key to attaining the target of 'health for all by the year 2000' (WHO 1979) and, with that target in mind, whether or not the health problems of any one nation could be significantly reduced by a conventional system of Western medicine was brought into question.

The epidemiology of developed nations is characterized by the diseases of affluence, by various forms of handicap, and by the growing incidence of diseases related to the aging process; and, hence, displays a rather different disease and demographic profile to that observed in developing countries. Yet the critique of primary health care when it is conceived largely as medical care is a universal one. As Kaprio (1979) remarked, in the context of Europe though with global relevance:

It is clear that technology, the primacy of the hospital, and excessive specialisation can only be reasonably attacked when they start to detract from a more holistic and effective appproach to care; when, for example, focusing attention on the hospital causes wastage of human resources, destroys continuity of care, costs more than simpler ways of improving health, and removes preventive medicine, other forms of community development and the consumer from the caring scene.

In the specific context of the developing world, many of the basic tenets of primary health care have, of course, been discussed, promoted and in a number of cases implemented as national policies for many years. One such example is India, where it is clear that the 'concept' was recognized early on. The Health Survey and Planning Committee was established in 1944 and recommended the development of a network of primary health centres from which primary health services, providing both curative and preventive care, would radiate through subcentres over the countryside, covering the entire population (Bhore Committee 1946). The result today is that about 5500 centres and 38 000 sub-centres now exist, each covering a population of 80 000 to 125 000 persons (Jagdish 1981). Such facilities, called basic health services in some countries, provide the necessary basis for the implementation of current notions of primary health care. As a signatory to the Alma Ata Declaration, the Government of India committed itself further to take steps to provide 'health for all' by moving towards having one health centre for every 50 000 persons by the year 2000 (WHO/IND 1980).

Why has the concept of primary health care assumed such world-wide prominence in current thinking, and what are the ideas that have influenced this choice of health strategy? Historically, apart from the extension of various public health measures in developing countries, the distribution of health services has been biased in favour of hospitals located in urban areas, and services have concentrated on the 'repair' aspects of health care. Disillusionment with expensive hospital-based and hospital-oriented medical services, and medical approaches to illness, have certainly been factors behind the growing concern about the inappropriateness of such services in the developing world, and the inability of such institutions to reach out to the basic health needs of rural populations and the urban poor. For instance, over 78 per cent of India's population is settled in rural areas, in approximately 576 000 villages, nearly half of which have a population of 500 or less. In addition, 39 per cent of its urban population live in cities with over half a million inhabitants, compared with 26 per cent twenty years ago (World Bank 1981).

Allied to this concern about over-medicalization, the underserved rural areas, and rapid urbanization in the developing world, are the interrelated issues of population growth and poverty. Many developing countries are characterized by high fertility rates and low birth spacing intervals. Again to cite India, it has a population of some 659 million (1979 estimates) and this figure is expected to increase to about 975 million by the year 2000. Put most simply and yet forcibly, children in the age band 0–14 years already constitute a little over 40 per cent of India's population. One of the oft-cited explanations about poor countries' slow rate of economic development and low per capita expenditure on health is that improvements in economic growth have been quickly dissipated by increases in population. As Chapter 2 discusses, population growth can be considered *a priori* to have both favourable and unfavourable effects on economic development (and vice versa).

In terms of poverty, national data disguises quite wide differences between urban and rural areas (and within urban areas) in many, if not most, of the widely used social indicators of quality of life. For example, it has been estimated in India, using caloric consumption as a guide, that 48 per cent of the rural and 41 per cent of the urban population were living below the poverty line. The death rate in 1977 was estimated to be 14.7 per thousand, with a marked disparity between rural and urban areas, which were 16 and 9.4 respectively. While overall infant mortality was 129 per thousand (in 1977), it was 139 in rural areas as against 80 per thousand in urban areas. Less than ten per cent of the population in rural areas of India today have proper sanitation or a protected water supply; 100 000 rural villages are without potable drinking water (Ramalingaswami 1981).

To these indices, which can be observed to a greater or lesser extent in many other developing countries, can be added a further point about the relationship between health and development. According to one recent source (Walt and Vaughan 1981), the current emphasis upon primary health care can be seen partly as a reaction against the earlier neglect of health in policies on development. Any government is necessarily concerned with seeking an appropriate balance between investment and consumption. In other words, it must determine what resources should be subtracted from immediate consumption, and invested to permit future higher levels of consumption. Early development theories have become increasingly criticized for their overriding preoccupation with investment in the physical (or material) elements of national growth, thereby viewing health and other social services as constituent members of a largely non-productive, consumption sector, only to be afforded once the vital investment needs had been met. In short, the role given to health in development policies centres on the degree to which 'health care' is viewed as an 'investment' rather than as a 'consumption' good. If the latter, then if agriculture is undeveloped, and industry is undeveloped, the economy will be expected to spare only limited amounts of resources for health services. If the former, then health services, along with other social sectors, will be expected to form part of an integrated inter-sectoral package to raise levels of socioeconomic development.

Definitions and concepts

Examination of the underlying causes for the primary health care movement is confused by a further difficulty that exists throughout the world: namely that the term 'primary health care' means different things to different people. Indeed, at present, though an international definition exists, it is not universally used or implemented. The meaning of the term has changed over time, originally being applied simply to primary medical care (the contribution of doctors outside hospitals) and community health services (the contribution of health workers also outside the hospital setting). Thus, general medical practitioners have traditionally been seen as the primary care providers in the United Kingdom, and so have various types of auxiliaries in many developing countries. As a result, in many countries in the world today, categories of health care are distinguished first and foremost in terms of the levels at which care is provided. Accordingly, one sees primary health care defined as treatment based in a health clinic, dispensary, or health centre close to where people live and work; secondary care as somewhat more specialized care based in fairly large community or district hospitals; and tertiary care as highly specialized, often technologically based, intensive care, centralized in large medical centres and commonly located in universities.

Not everyone, however, has been content with this classification, not least for its neglect of health-related activities. Its virtue is that it is administratively tidy but, in the context of many developing countries, may disguise the many overlapping services that are provided by different levels of care. This raises the question of whether or not primary health care might be better defined and analysed in terms of what it offers, rather than how it is presently structured. Indeed, this is the basis on which the WHO definition is composed. In terms of what primary health care might encompass, the Alma Ata Declaration offered a much more far-reaching philosophy than the traditional definition, by stating that at least the following components should be included:

Education concerning prevailing health problems and the methods of preventing and controlling them; promotion of food supply and proper nutrition; an adequate supply of safe water and basic sanitation; maternal and child health care, including family planning; immunisation against the major infectious diseases; prevention and control of locally endemic diseases; appropriate treatment of common diseases and injuries; and provision of essential drugs.

This definition was underlined by five criteria that distinguished it from the earlier and often narrower conception of primary health care: equitable distribution; community involvement; focus on prevention; appropriate technology; and a multi-sectoral approach. Hence, the terms should be viewed in a rather more rigorous and all-embracing form than the activities of some of its practitioners might imply:

Primary health care has been seen by some as simply the use of community health workers from a poor rural locality, trained to do their best with the over-simplified tools at their disposal. Others believe it to be a new name for the expansion in coverage of the old 'basic health services' where curative care was provided to passive recipients. Another view is that it is a combination of the activities known as the 'eight components' of primary health care included in the Declaration of Alma Ata. Finally, it is also thought of as an independent system, having no ties to other health services. If we look at primary health care in any of these ways, then it becomes a second-rate service for the poor and rural areas, and this means in practice the consolidation of social injustice in the field of health (Tejada-de-Rivero 1981).

Support for primary health care defined in terms of what it offers is evident in a review of 33 definitions of 'primary health care' (Ruby, Vpahurch, and Weisfeld 1977). Eight characteristics were mentioned repeatedly: accessibility, comprehensiveness, co-ordination, continuity, first contact, quality, management, and community involvement. Arguably, therefore, what differentiated primary health care from other forms of care was to be explained in terms of these common characteristics. For instance, 'continuity' and 'co-ordination' appeared in over 70 per cent of the definitions studied, doubtless reflecting a widespread view that primary health care be seen not only as the point of entry to health care, but also as bearing prime responsibility for promoting health and rendering appropriate care. Further, these definitions were couched in terms that were comprehensive enough to include the activities of a wide range of health workers.

As WHO has recognized, any strategy which purports to be comprehensive should assess the primary health services programme alongside other health-related socioeconomic programmes. (For instance, in India, the Integrated Rural Development Programme, Nutrition Programme, Integrated Child Development Scheme, and National Adult Education Programme, have all been launched in recent years by Ministries/Departments of the Government other than the Ministry of Health and Family Welfare.) For the same reason, a comprehensive approach should include consideration of the roles of traditional healers, voluntary workers, and private practitioners who may offer alternative or complementary services to those of government-supported or financed primary health services (for instance, again from India, with schoolteachers, *dais* (traditional midwives), housewives, and village practitioners who use other than the 'Western' or allopathic systems of medicine).

Not everyone, however, will accept this somewhat idealized concept of primary health care, nor will they agree that it is reflected in actual practice. In consequence, it does appear likely that developing countries will continue to use a range of definitions and concepts of primary health care which stress specific aspects of its purpose, structure, and function. Recognizing this fact, this chapter intends to work within its own guideline; namely, to concentrate its attention upon those aspects of primary health care considered to lie within the remit of Western and indigenous medical and health services, though not to the total exclusion of those health-related activities considered important influences on health, such as sanitation and water supply. To focus upon primary health care defined in this way is not to assume that health needs are solely, or even predominantly, met by a network of primary health services. Rather, the assumption underlying this chapter is that these services do have an important contribution to make to health and that it is pertinent to analyse—from an economic perspective—the resource and cost implications of their delivery.

Financial and cost aspects

Defined in the above terms, primary health care in most developing countries is provided by a variety of organizations, public, private, and voluntary. Any study of primary health care financing, therefore, has to distinguish between the sources of finance and the health care institutions responsible for spending: the health agency that spends the money may not be the agency that raises it or distributes it. However, it is widely recognized that a substantial information gap on health expenditures exists in most developing countries. The data that are available cover mainly government health expenditures and health budgets, often at an aggregate level, and the information is not structured to provide data on the cost and financial aspects of primary health care *per se* (see Chapter 3).

Hence, a prior task is to define carefully the reasons for collecting any additional financial and cost data for carrying out specific cost analyses. Since primary health care has been widely accepted as an approach to achieve the goal of health for all by the year 2000, national, regional, or local studies on the financing and costing of primary health care may be undertaken for a number of reasons, including the following:

(1) to explore the possibility of developing new financial *sources* for primary health care, or of extending existing sources;
(2) to examine what communities are *contributing*, and different population groups (classified by age, sex, income) are *paying*, towards the cost of primary health care, and how this compares with the volume and the value of services they receive;
(3) to identify and measure the *cost* of delivering primary health care and the

resource requirements (manpower, facilities, drugs, etc.) of any proposed changes in forms of delivery (the objective being either to determine low-cost ways of providing primary services or to contain overall costs within specified resource constraints); and

(4) to examine the determinants of the demand for, and utilization of, primary health care, with the objective of influencing these to obtain a more equit-able distribution.

These are important issues for national planners, local managers, community organizations, and members of the general public and, hence, are now con-sidered separately below.

Sources of finance

Conventionally, when identifying the financing sources for primary health care, a distinction is drawn between public (and quasi-public) monies and private sources of funds (WHO 1978*b*). Thus:

Public (and quasi-public) sources	*Private sources*
(1) General tax revenue	(1) Private health insurance
(2) Deficit financing	(2) Employer-financed services
(3) Earmarked taxes	(3) Charitable and voluntary contributions
(4) Social insurance	(4) Community self-help and fund-raising
(5) Local tax revenues	(5) Private household expenditure
(6) State-run lotteries and betting	

At a national level, developing countries will fall into recognizable groups in terms of the balance between private and public sources, and between reliance on tax revenues (national or local) or on health insurance payments. However, as more than one Report has acknowledged (WHO 1978*a*), for developing countries to rely solely on systems of financing health care that are current in more affluent countries will be as unwise as to rely on the technology practised in those countries. Specifically, covering the cost of primary health care through national taxation may be quite impracticable in poor, predominantly agricultural societies.

In consequence, financing is likely to be a combined effort relying on multiple sources. At the local level, sources of funding will be drawn from the following:

(1) individuals (family plus relatives, including incomes remitted from abroad);
(2) communities;
(3) local insurance schemes;
(4) local industry or agricultural enterprises or co-operatives;
(5) charity/religious missions;
(6) State or regional revenues;
(7) Central government revenues; and
(8) external assistance.

The number of sources, and levels of resources generated, may vary from one locality to another, with respect both to the per capita amount and the proportion raised locally. The greater the reliance on local fund-raising, the more likely will be disparities in the level and quality of primary health care available in different parts of any one country and, other things being equal, in the quality of people's health.

Community involvement and payments by individuals

In the circumstances that are likely to prevail in the developing world, an important factor will therefore be the extent of the community's sharing of the costs of primary health care, either in the form of money or contributions in kind. Many examples exist where communities have shared with government (and individuals) the responsibility for providing in cash (or kind) resources towards primary health care; though often few details are known about the amounts, distribution, and utilization of such resources. However, as Djukanovic and Mach argue (1975), the issue of community involvement is not one confined to finance:

Financing and decision-making are complementary functions that reinforce each other; they place the community in a position of authority as it shoulders responsibility for its own services. In countries where this is the national approach, community leaders are well aware of local health problems. They understand the role, scope and potential of their primary health care service, and they take an active interest in its management. What is more, the health institution at the level nearest to primary care is clearly more alert to the community's needs and wishes (p. 99).

Not surprisingly, perhaps, experience to date has revealed that while the policy expounded above is commendable, its implementation is beset with difficulties. Included in the Report of an inter-regional workshop (WHO/UNICEF 1980) was a summary of country statements about community responsibilities for financing primary health care. Two examples are cited here, those of Ethiopia and Kenya. In 1978 the Ministry of Health, Ethiopia, began the training of community health agents (CHAs). Initially, the farmers' organizations and urban dwellers' associations were to be partly responsible for the training costs of the CHA (food, lodging, and stationery), and subsequently for the full costs of the services later provided by those trained (drugs, equipment, and salary, if any). In Kenya, the introduction of a community health worker scheme (CHW) envisaged the community's participation in the selection of its CHWs, in contributing labour and local materials to improve water supplies and, most significantly, in cash contributions for the support of CHWs.

As in all similar community-financed schemes, much depends upon both the *ability* and the *willingness* of the local community to continue to provide permanent funds for health workers. No details were presented on this point for Ethiopia, but in Kenya it appeared that a major problem was the difficulty of sustaining the expected level of financial support for the CHW. Although originally intended to be a part-time worker (rather like the 'barefoot doctor'), the demand for CHW services was said to be such as to require more-or-less full-time work. The inadequate compensation to the CHWs for lost hours of work was apparently considered to be a major factor leading to CHW disillusionment. It had been expected that sufficient monies would have been generated from the initial cash contributions by households, to be followed by a 'fee-for-service' system of payments, but community resistance to fee schedules had meant that this was realized only in part.

It is, therefore, important to study the consequences of any changes in methods of financing health care in terms of the extent to which they encourage or discourage developments in primary health care. For instance, as demonstrated in Kenya, a key policy issue is the role to be played by direct consumer charges, deductibles and co-payments. Even in primary health care, it is unlikely that services will always be provided free of charge, without limit on usage and time. More likely, restrictions will be (and are) imposed either in terms of *coverage* (according to criteria of income, source of employment, etc.) or in terms of cost *ceilings* (based on fee or tariff schedules). Part of the rationale for these restrictions stems from a concern that to make health services totally free of charge seriously constrains their expansion and development. For instance, in Bangladesh (Choudhury 1981) some means of pricing health care is seen to be appropriate and necessary to generate resources and finance health services. In developing countries generally, some of these means are based on payment for items received, usually drugs. Fees received from the sale of drugs (or the difference between fees and the cost price) may then be employed for payments to community health workers or for other health-related activities. Another means is to base contributions upon actual usage of services, so that a large proportion of the costs of primary health care is met by the payment of consumer charges.

It cannot be ignored that some of those in favour of making increasing use of such charges do so on ideological grounds. They consider that the promotion of a pricing policy in the primary health care field presents an opportunity for the community in general, and individuals in particular, to 'participate' in the allocation of resources by signalling their preferences to providers and decision-makers. They further argue that individuals should be encouraged to consume only that quantity of primary health care for which the perceived benefits exceeds the cost of the resources used. Hence, they hope the financial impact would be twofold: to raise revenue and affect favourably the behaviour of consumers towards 'economy' in usage.

The counter-argument is provided by those who wish to give all individuals, regardless of income, class, sex, or race, equal access to primary health care. To do so, they believe, implies service payments that are unrelated to actual usage, or no payment at all. Certainly, the provision of primary health care free at the point of consumption (or at less than cost) will change the way in which the cost-benefit of such services is distributed among the population (Lee 1982). It may, for instance, redistribute income. It may also change the use that different sections of the population make of the services.

Paradoxically, it could be argued that charges, if used selectively, could effect a more equitable utilization of health care throughout the country, both spatially and between population groups. An illustrative example is offered by Gish (1975), who argues the case for introducing charges at the out-patient departments of urban hospitals but not at rural dispensaries. The major objective of such a policy would not be to raise revenue but rather to move towards an improved distribution of services. The means would be selective (hospital) charges to restrain the relative over-utilization of such services by those who enjoy the easiest access to them; the ends would be a re-alignment of resources to those considered most in need.

More generally, whether or not charges should be made for primary health care and, if so, for what services and at what levels, are hotly disputed issues (see also Chapter 7). It is worth noting that requiring cash payments or relating fees to incomes where incomes are mainly derived in kind from subsistence agriculture is not always feasible, and the administration of such a system may be beyond the capacity of these countries. Furthermore, there may well be categories of primary care that should be exempted from charges and financed entirely from public funds (for instance, preventive and promotive health care), especially where these benefit the whole community, not just those individuals directly affected (such as the provision of potable water, the protection of dwellings against insects and rodents, and community health education).

Costs and resources

The developing world is characterized by a multitude of different health care systems, in which the primary care situation and its sources of funding differ materially from setting to setting. What is common to all settings, however, is that there are limits to the amounts a government, community, or individual feels able to allocate to primary health care. Hence, in determining a pattern of primary health care appropriate to local circumstances, an important economic factor is 'cost' since this will determine whether a given approach is feasible or not within present resource constraints. Costs are incurred both by the *producers* of health services, through their use of staff, buildings, equipment, materials, supplies, and by *consumers*, who use their own time to seek and receive primary care, who incur transport costs, and who spend money on drugs, fees, etc. In short: primary health care imposes costs on both sides, in terms of foregone opportunities to use the resources in other ways.

It follows that to evaluate how well finite resources (human and financial) are being used, it is necessary to link together the sources of finance with the categories of expenditure, in order to link both these against the purposes of such income and expenditure. Yet, although the methodology does exist to complete this task (see Chapter 3), needs are often quantified (if at all) in epidemiological terms and resources in budgeting or manpower terms, with no easy way of relating one set of data to the other. Hence, a means is required of expressing the major categories of primary health care expenditure in relation to the components of primary health care. One example where this approach was adopted is the Narangwal Rural Health Centre Project in India. The methodology involved collecting minimal information using, as a bridging mechanism between needs and resources, a grid of (eleven) specific functions being performed in rural health centres, along the dimensions of the time spent and the cost for each function, and the morbidity being treated (Taylor *et al.* 1976). This method of functional analysis has now been adapted and used in studies in Nepal, Bangladesh, Iran, Egypt, Nigeria, and many more countries (Taylor 1980). In essence, the idea is to analyse the use of resources by the various purposes they serve, and to relate resources used to results achieved, or to outputs that can be measured.

Access, coverage, and utilization

It is important that information about the sources of finance for, and the costs of, primary health services should also be linked with information both on the coverage of the population served, and on the take-up and utilization of such services. By doing so, questions can be answered about those features of primary health care which appear to affect the take-up and use of services, and about why there are groups within the population for whom difficulties of access and coverage appear to exist.

It is helpful at this stage to identify the processes by which an individual's demands for health care are, or are not, matched by supply (see Fig. 5.1). To

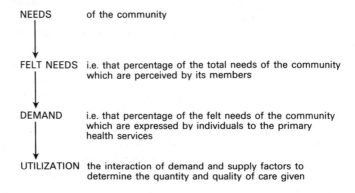

Fig. 5.1. Demand, supply, and the utilization of primary health care.

consider the individual first, he has to perceive that his actual health status is, or is likely to be, less than his desired health status—now, or in the future. This perception of *felt* need leads to his first decision, whether to seek help or not. If he decides to do something, other than waiting for the illness to occur or, if the illness has occurred, for it to cure itself, then he examines the modes and choices available. These might include, for example, self-medication using his own family's remedies; seeking advice and buying the products of the nearest village store-keeper or pharmacist; seeking assistance from traditional healers; or seeking advice from the government's primary health services.

In any of these cases, by acting, he translates his felt need into *demand*. Looking in particular at the last of these cases, it is important to discover and understand:

(1) the factors that caused the individual to consult the primary health services; and

(2) the factors determining the response made by those services to this person's demand (Lee 1979).

A number of factors will affect whether or not a person seeks access to primary health care. Attempts have been made to tease out the processes by which people not only label themselves as 'in need' (felt need), but also actively seek primary health care (demand). The same vector of conditions will not apply to all persons, but among those that can be listed are the following: methods of payment used; costs incurred; distance and travel time; means of transport; administrative barriers; professional attitudes; cultural and social barriers between health workers and patients; confidence in, or fear of, sophisticated technology and know-how; and attitudes to illness rooted in the cultural pattern of the community. Ironically, even where primary health services are provided for the community, these factors may combine to ensure that the services are under-utilized. Ideally, as can be readily agreed, accessibility to primary health care implies that it should be geographically, financially, culturally, and function-ally within easy reach of the whole community in rural as much as in urban settings (WHO 1978*a*).

Indeed, as this indicates, utilization will necessarily be affected as much by the characteristics and supply of services, as by the characteristics of consumers. It is clear from estimates that probably four-fifths of the world's population, living mainly in rural areas and urban slums, have no access to any continuing form of health care (WHO 1978*a*). Whether due to the past inequitable development of services (for instance, by colonial governments), lack of political commit-ment, lack of resources, inefficient organization and management, or other reasons, resources when made available have often been monopolized by the more vocal and demanding section of the population, namely the well-established and relatively richer urban populations.

This concentration of resources within the urban areas, and upon the urban elite, demonstrates that it is necessary to disentangle issues of rich and poor from those of geographical location. As Walt and Vaughan (1981) remark:

There has been, up to now, a strange neglect of the peri-urban and urban poor who make up an increasing percentage of many developing countries' popula-tions. People who work in cement factories, but live in *favelas*, under shanty roofs, without electric light or sewerage systems, with stand pipes down the road, who walk miles into work, or are squashed into poor and overcrowded transport, may be worse off than their rural cousins.

Economic agglomerations of urban poor will be a continuing characteristic of the future. For much of the world's poor, it is argued that the city offers the only hope for survival, and so:

> whether they are right or not, whether they stay or whether they return to be replaced by others, whether they come in desperation or whether they come as 'pioneers'—they continue to come (England 1978).

At the present time, however, few primary health services are located in the high density slums where they could be argued to be most needed, and the problems for the poor and destitute of actually being seen at an urban hospital and of securing a hospital bed may be quite substantial. For the rural population, physical access to far-off secondary or tertiary care can be a considerable problem and rural primary health services are often the only services which are accessible and available.

Alternative approaches and appropriate technologies

It would be difficult to claim that a great deal is known about the relative efficiency or cost-effectiveness of alternative approaches to preventing or treating the diseases of the developing world. For the most part, the answers are simply not known, and evaluation in primary health care has been largely undertaken as a descriptive approach, describing inputs and processes, not measuring costs, outputs, and outcomes. Most important of all, what are the *opportunity costs* of providing such services? Under what conditions is it more appropriate to focus resources on risk factors common to many illnesses—on poverty, malnutrition, sanitation, water supply—rather than on medical services?

Evaluation demands an examination of the costs and benefits of alternative broad strategies as much as an examination of particular technologies. In this regard, what underlies the supply of any good or service—and primary health care is no exception—is its *production function*. The production function identifies the technical relation between the output of that service and the resources (or inputs) used to produce it. Hence, which techniques for improving health will be the most appropriate techniques depends both on the cost of each type of care, and on their relative *effectiveness*. For example, the difference in the cost (training cost and salary) of putting to work a doctor and health auxiliary must be compared to differences in their productivities. For a wide range of common ailments, the difference in the effectiveness of treatment between a doctor and an auxiliary is much less than the difference in the costs of their training and present levels of remuneration.

It follows that a careful study of substitution possibilities is called for, both between different forms of health worker (e.g. doctor, auxiliary, community health volunteer) and between labour and capital resources. Such a study will have to be related first and foremost to the country's infrastructure and, in the short run at least, to the relative availability of different forms of manpower. Moreover, if the objective of 'primary health care for all' is to be attained, it will require not only a critical review of manpower requirements, but also of present methods, techniques, equipment, and drug prescribing in primary health care, and a critique of the locations in which services are, or could be, provided.

As has already been noted, the level of technology adopted in much of the developing world is one that is costly, capital-intensive, and ill-adapted to local needs, requiring a set of highly trained personnel to operate services. The consequence is that services are not only inequitably distributed but also inefficiently provided, offering 'health for a few' instead of 'health for all'. It can be argued that what is needed is to modify or replace that technology so that it is less costly, more labour-intensive, well-adapted to local needs, and utilizes to the full local resources, knowledge, and skills.

In short, what is needed is 'appropriate health technology'. The word 'technology' means any association of methods, techniques, and equipment which, together with human resources, addresses a health problem. 'Appropriate' means that, besides being scientifically sound, the technology is also acceptable to those who apply it and to those for whom it is provided. 'Appropriate' also means treating people in their situation (urban conurbation or small village) in the least-cost but most effective way consistent with the severity of their problem. It follows that at the primary care level the development of health technologies should focus on simple, least-cost, and self-reliant measures. To illustrate the direct relevance to developing countries of this concept of appropriate health technology, ideas are drawn from two sources: the first of water supply and sanitation in India; the second of drug prescribing in Mozambique.

Examples of innovative methods of improving water supply and sanitation in India, based on appropriate technologies, were suggested at a Regional WHO Workshop held in New Delhi in 1980 (WHO/SEARO 1980). Ideas generated included the:

(1) manufacture and testing of different kinds of hand pumps made from local materials;
(2) development of rainwater-collecting cisterns, again with locally available materials;
(3) development of simple methods of removing turbidity of surface water;
(4) iodinizer for pond water sterilization to be used with a hand pump;
(5) involvement of the community in setting up individual and public water supply and sanitation facilities;
(6) development of simple and easily maintained privies useful in areas where water was scarce;
(7) development of ventilated pit latrines; and,
(8) development of latrine and kitchen waste-disposal measures in water stagnant areas.

The second example is drawn from the health services of Mozambique (Barker, Marzagao, and Segall 1980) which, in 1977, spent 20 per cent of its budget on pharmaceutical products. Proportionally, this was the second largest category of expenditure (salaries being the main category); but if each citizen had received an equal share, it approximated to only two-thirds of a single US dollar per capita each year. Concern over the drugs bill *in toto* was attributed to two factors: the opportunity cost of that expenditure in terms of resources that were retained inside the hospital setting; and the high imports bill for pharmaceuticals and the consequential drain upon the country's valuable foreign currency reserves.

In order to help health workers prescribe more economically and no less effectively, a list was prepared from which examples are cited below, illustrating how it is possible to treat patients with simple and inexpensive drugs, and to restrict the prescription of expensive preparations to the relatively few situations where they are considered really necessary:

(1) liquid preparations (syrups, drops) are much more expensive than tablets or capsules of the same drug—for many drugs, the liquid preparations were shown to be 2-20 times more expensive than the solid products;
(2) because of their expense, multivitamin products should never be given as placebos, especially in liquid form;
(3) injections are frequently much more expensive than the same drug given by mouth—for a range of drugs, injections cost 3-20 times more than the same dose given by mouth;
(4) when a patient has an upper respiratory infection, it is questionable whether an antibiotic is really required;
(5) co-trimoxazole can be replaced by tetracycline, at a greatly reduced cost.

The authors argued that a question to be asked at all times of those prescribing drugs is first, does the patient really need any medicine at all and, if yes, would a cheaper one do as well or nearly as well? The criteria of 'cheapness' and 'effectiveness' are not, however, always easy to assess, especially when they require a trade-off between them. For example, while tablets may be cheaper than injections, the advantages of injections relative to tablets are: the dose is received immediately (the patient may not purchase his prescription for tablets); the dose is administered without requiring subsequent action by the patient (the tablets may be forgotten); and the dose is the correct measure (some of the tablets may be sold or given to another person). However, putting these questions can help countries identify effective drugs at a low cost for primary health care, and seek low-cost methods of production and distribution.

The overall question of appropriate technology is not confined solely to the issue of *what* to provide, but also of *where* to provide appropriate care. The further people live from a health facility, the less likely they are to attend unless their need is very great, and populations which do not have a health centre or dispensary near to hand may not receive Westernized medicine at all. As a result, the effect of distance—or, rather, distance and travel time—is an important consideration in the equitable distribution of health facilities and in their take-up, especially in rural areas.

As Sorkin (1976), among others, has noted, there are at least two important reasons why take-up is negatively related to distance and time. First, the greater the distance to a health facility, the higher the transport cost to the patient and any relatives who may accompany him. Secondly, other things being equal, it takes more time to travel a longer distance. As the opportunity cost of time is positive (taking the form, for instance, of foregone agricultural work and/or income), people will be reluctant to travel great distances because of the significant opportunity cost involved. Hence, such travel may only be undertaken when illness is perceived to be extremely serious and when all locally available possibilities for care are exhausted, and sometimes not even then.

Consideration has therefore been given to designing innovative forms of delivering stationary and mobile health care services which address the health problems of communities, especially in rural areas. Mobile health teams in particular have been the subject of much debate on questions such as: (1) economy—are they worth the money?; (2) manpower—are they a proper use of skilled personnel?; (3) what is the best way to run them? (Cox 1969). In practice, most of these questions can only be answered at the local level and the answers are dependent upon a number of factors such as the topography and geography of the population, the hoped-for types of health care to be provided, and the costs and benefits of alternative forms of care.

First, the geographical setting and the patterns of rural settlement will be relevant. Populations may be scattered or concentrated in villages, and the villages may be scattered or concentrated in particular areas. Geographical terrains vary from the mountainous to the relatively flat. Road systems and public transport systems, likewise, will be of varying quantity and quality, and may be affected by climatic conditions. Secondly, mobile units can usually visit particular locations only periodically, and are likely to be inappropriate where continuity of care is important (Gish and Walker 1977). However, some health services, such as pre-natal and well baby care, immunizations and health education, can be offered periodically—and, hence, are strong candidates for mobile care. Depending upon the density of the population, road conditions, and distances to be travelled, a mobile team based at the district health centre might travel continuously or for some period of time, or it might return each night to the district headquarters.

It follows that the whole question of appropriate mobile services is not a straightforward one. Moreover, it can become entangled with professional values. There are those health workers who resist any efforts directed towards the development of mobile services because of alleged difficulties in achieving professional 'standards' of health care. This view could be misplaced, given that the alternative for rural communities may be no care at all. At the other extreme, there are those who would travel any distance, at any cost, in order to reach the very last villager. Such an approach may also be misplaced, on grounds of both practicality and of cost.

A number of principles of general interest emerge from this discussion. First, and perhaps most generally, there are usually more ways of carrying out a health programme than tend conventionally to be considered as options in health planning, and these alternatives will involve some trade-off between cost and effectiveness. This leads on to the second point. In choosing between the various ways of delivering health care, what are important are the costs and benefits at the *margin*. For instance, in most immunization programmes, once those children within easy reach have been immunized, a higher yield (i.e. greater coverage) can usually be obtained only at a higher cost per child immunized. This is illustrated graphically in Fig. 5.2, where the total cost is shown to increase appreciably as one tries to immunize the whole population. At the same time, as the diagram also illustrates, the rate of cost increase (i.e. marginal cost) is likely to differ between strategies.

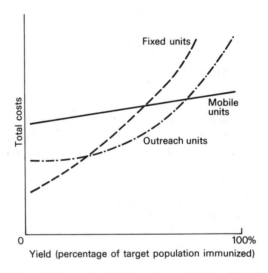

Fig. 5.2. The relative costs of alternative methods of immunization.

The marginal cost concept is of wide application to both strategic planning and local management issues (Creese 1979). Where, for example, the cost of using stationary plus outreach services leads to escalating marginal costs per fully immunized child—as when very small numbers of children are being immunized in a full day's work by a primary health team—it becomes important to consider the possibility of alternative strategies. If populations are widely scattered, so that an outreach team which returns each evening to the district headquarters has to spend a disproportionate amount of time travelling, then it may become more cost-effective to immunize these sections of the population by means of a fully mobile service. By referring to Fig. 5.3, it is possible to determine the best (i.e. optimum) combination of approaches by identifying the threshold at which it becomes cheaper to immunize the extra child by

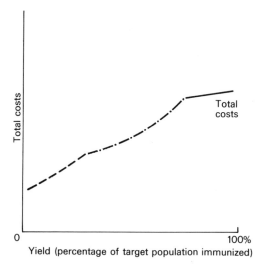

Fig. 5.3. The optimum mix of immunization methods.

mobile rather than by outreach services, and when either strategy is to be preferred to stationary units. (Necessarily, the cost per immunized child in isolated rural communities will be much higher than in densely populated urban communities. In addition, therefore, to issues of cost-effectiveness are questions of equity, which are explored in detail in Chapter 8.)

Health manpower resources

Types of health manpower vary between and within countries according to, for instance, the population's needs, the resources available for satisfying them, historical traditions, and the power of different professional groups. It should not be ignored, however, that many types of manpower are, or could be, potential substitutes for each other, in both technical and financial terms. Indeed, the presence in many countries of doctors, paramedicals, professionally trained nurses, family health workers, health auxiliaries, and community health volunteers, as well as traditional practitioners and birth attendants, suggests that the opportunity already exists to seek to adjust their absolute numbers, their roles, and their mix, as well as their methods of payment, to a pattern of manpower use appropriate to primary health care.

The point about substitutability, now generally accepted and a concept familiar to economists, is that in many areas of primary health care, people with a limited training, appropriate for tackling the major local health problems, can function very well as alternatives to medical practitioners. For instance, for some time now, the use of various local health workers such as health auxiliaries, and more recently community health volunteers, has been advocated as a means both of improving the community's access to basic and primary health care and of increasing the actual amounts of care received. Indeed, these workers are not only perceived to be the point of first or early contact with health care, but in practical terms may well be the only regular contact. Though health manpower planners would perhaps refer to the lack of a clear world-wide consensus about the roles and respective merits of these, and other, categories of health worker, in relation to appropriate technologies they do once again indicate the potential scope for viewing some imaginative and innovative forms of health worker as real options.

The concept of the 'health auxiliary', however, has been subject to varying interpretations. An auxiliary has conventionally been defined as a person who is paid to assist and be supervised by a professional worker and, hence, both complements and supplements professional staff. Most would not now define the parameters of the job description in such narrow terms, and believe that auxiliary workers exhibit a degree of independence of thought and action that is not captured by this definition. Indeed, the term 'auxiliary' is now out of fashion, though the often claimed benefits of employing that type of health worker in the primary health care field can still be listed as follows:

(1) they overcome or reduce the acute shortage of professionally trained staff in rural areas where doctors are reluctant or unwilling to practise;
(2) they can be trained less expensively than professionals;
(3) they are remunerated at a much lower level;
(4) they are no less effective or perhaps better at carrying out a range of duties (especially routine tasks);
(5) they are closer to the people they serve, physically and socially; and
(6) they enable doctors to concentrate on extending their specialist skills to larger populations.

The basis and the strength of such services lies in a cadre of suitably selected and trained primary health workers: the real issue is not therefore doctors or auxiliaries, but what kind and mix of health workers are most appropriate and how might health manpower planning be most appropriately conducted (see, for instance, Chapter 6).

There is little doubt that the Chinese Cultural Revolution (1966–76) re-focused and, in some cases, revolutionized professional views on manpower for the delivery of primary health care. A reliance upon professional medical services was at least temporarily abandoned and replaced by the 'barefoot doctor' and volunteer health aide. Barefoot doctors were farm workers trained in simple diagnostic and treatment techniques; they gave simple medical care or advice, but they also continued to do farm work. Admittedly, the term was a misnomer because they were seldom barefoot (save in the rice paddies), and were certainly not doctors in the professional sense of the term. Rather they were essentially agricultural workers and were paid as such, notwithstanding that they gave at least a part of their time to health work in health stations or in the fields (e.g. providing health education and preventive medicine, and dealing with medical emergencies). In contrast, health aides worked during their lunch hour or after their regular work and were not paid for this service (Sidel and Sidel 1980).

Similar developments have subsequently taken place elsewhere in the world. For instance in Thailand, the promotion of the community volunteer is seen as an important approach to developing community participation, through the training of village volunteers and village health communicators (WHO/UNICEF 1980). The village volunteer is trained to provide simple first-aid and basic care of minor ailments, to advise about family planning, to refer more serious cases of illness, supervise communicators, and co-ordinate local government health activities. A parallel development in Bangladesh envisages the major facilities for primary health care to be a health complex in each rural location, with an auxiliary cadre of paid health workers raised for each village, in addition to volunteer village health workers selected and trained to work in their own communities (Choudhury 1981).

The funding possibilities for primary health workers (including urban as well as rural health auxiliaries, and village health workers at the community level) are numerous. There may be village support on a fee-for-service basis, or local government support from local taxation or central government grant. The community workers may be part-time volunteers or they may sell medicines or be supported by a surcharge collected from patients at district health centres or hospitals. Or, if funds are forthcoming, the government may assume responsibility for their entire salaries (Smith 1982). Whichever method or combination of methods is decided upon, the issue of remuneration for the various categories of health worker will continue to be an important one—for it might prove extremely difficult for developing countries to rely extensively upon recruiting community health workers on a largely unpaid and voluntary basis, since the opportunity cost of their time is unlikely to be zero.

While these new and innovative types of manpower are emerging, it should not be forgotten that practitioners of traditional medicine, including traditional birth attendants, not only exist but in rural areas may still comprise about 90 per cent of the primary health care workers (broadly defined). It has been estimated, indeed, that traditional medicine is the principal, if not the only, source of medical care for two-thirds of the world's population (Vuori 1982). Traditional medicine exists in many forms, and at various stages of development, ranging from formalized systems of indigenous medicine (e.g. Ayurvedic and Chinese medicine) to non-formalized traditional systems of medicine (e.g. herbalism, bone-setting, and spiritualism). Indeed, as Skeet and Elliott have observed (1978), two contrasting phenomena are often apparent in many rural areas of some developing countries. On the one hand, there is a lack of official health services and, yet, where they do exist they may be poorly used. Rather, the local population uses, and may even show a preference for, the services of traditional practitioners because they are well-integrated into their local communities. This is hardly surprising for they are a part of the 'community', its cultural heritage and traditions, and can exert considerable influence on local health practices.

It is also hardly surprising that efforts are now being made in a number of developing countries to incorporate both traditional healers and their remedies into the primary health care sector, to upgrade their skills or to train them as health auxiliaries and community health workers. These efforts do not deny the requirement that there be a careful analysis of the benefits of traditional medicine and the role of healers in society (Barker 1982). There is a tendency to look upon the traditional practitioner as an untapped resource for modern medicine rather than as an equal partner; the intended integration is to take place under conditions dictated by the modern system. The real issue, however, is how best to mobilize health manpower resources in *both* 'traditional' and 'modern' forms of medicine, and deploy them for effective delivery of primary health care, rather than necessarily seeing the answer in terms of additional funding for 'modern' health services (Fendall 1981).

Allied to the marked growth of enthusiasm to embrace the concept of health workers such as community volunteers, and to reinforce existing personnel with traditional healers, there also appears to be growing enthusiasm for the self-help and self-reliance movement. In large part, this enthusiasm is due to the encouragement given to it by governments and international agencies. Governments in particular can see that there are inherent benefits, both social and economic, in using the community and the individual as self-provider and self-financer of primary health care. For one thing, as has repeatedly been noted, most health care (especially in the rural setting) is carried out without professional medical intervention, so that people do already assume a great deal of responsibility for the diagnosis and treatment of themselves and their families. It is debatable, however, whether or not the self-help and community-help movements are attempting to make a virtue out of a necessity. Certainly, from an economic point of view, it is recognized that the individual, his family and his local community are potential resource sources for primary health care and may well be appropriate sources in cost-effective terms. Unquestionably, the community is the largest untapped source of labour for health promotion that is available to developing countries: one reason it remains untapped is due to a reluctance in some quarters to look further than 'modern' medicine to meet the community's needs for primary health care.

To those who propose a 'radical' model of primary health care, it is likely that their health system would operate mainly through community mechanisms. Rather than providing primary care directly, health personnel would focus increasingly on expanding the capacity of the community to solve its own problems. The argument would be that the health system would be 'on tap', rather than 'on top', to provide care where necessary. Therefore, primary health care would be handled mostly in the homes and villages and largely by community workers and volunteers. For many developing countries, the issue to be resolved is whether self-help, or a large and self-supported volunteer sector, is ever to be more than a fringe issue, given the position, importance and the status of those trained in the Western system of medicine; their influence on popular demands;

the present pyramid of professional medical power; the undoubted problems in organizing community participation; and the need for primary health care to be supported and supervised by the rest of the health system.

Summary and conclusion

Reproducing the most sophisticated of medical technologies is not only very costly and well beyond the capacities of most developing nations, it is now widely accepted as being misplaced. Rather, a strategy directed at Primary Health Care—to place 'appropriate' health services within reach of everyone—is considered increasingly to be an effective and equitable response to the needs of populations. Certainly, if primary health care were to be judged by the size of the literature devoted to it, then no-one could today fail to misjudge its importance. In contrast, the issue of how the primary health care approach is to be put into practice remains to be resolved. Despite enthusiasm throughout the world for primary health care, and the considerable literature devoted to it, few attempts have been made—from an economics standpoint—to analyse what it is and to determine what it can do, with what resources and at what cost.

This chapter has set out to identify and discuss a number of policy issues that are considered deserving of close attention. These can be summarized in terms of a set of questions which interested parties can ask of their policies and present services.

General
1. What is meant by the term 'primary health care' and what are the concepts incorporated in it?

Financing and expenditure
2. What are the sources of finance for primary health care, and to what extent is it possible to develop new sources (of resources and money) or extend existing ones?
3. What is the distribution of financing burdens between groups in the population?
4. How best can data on expenditure patterns be related to the purposes of that expenditure?

Need, demand, and utilization
5. What are the determinants of the demands being made upon primary health care?
6. What primary health services are provided to whom, why, and with what results in terms of equity?

Efficiency and effectiveness
7. What are the cost determinants of primary health care, and are they amenable to change and control by managers?
8. How will costs alter in response to changes in the size, content, and location of individual health programmes?
9. What opportunities exist for resource substitution (including manpower)

in the provision of primary health care, and what are the comparative productivities and relative costs of different resources?

10. Is there any marginal benefit from delivering primary health care versus not delivering it?

11. If so, can primary health care be organized to affect appreciably mortality and morbidity rates, or are these determined outside the field of primary health care, as presently defined?

Responses to these and similar questions could present a picture to health policy-makers and planners which indicates, for example, the range of work that can be expected from different types and levels of health worker, and at what cost; who does or does not use the primary health care services, and why; who is or is not referred to hospital, and by whom; and whether or not a greater investment in primary care will lead to reductions in the demand for secondary and tertiary care. It is clear that primary health care is a highly political issue, and that in all the above questions, governments, health workers, and the public will be likely to have their own objectives and perceptions. This leads to the conclusion that technical knowledge and political will should be closely linked. Economists, and those using economic concepts and techniques, will have to give close attention to the motivations of central policy-makers, local communities, and local managers, and considerable thought to devising appropriate structures in primary health care, and to adjusting the health technology to fit the resources available in the developing countries.

REFERENCES

Barker, C., Marzagao, C., and Segall, M. (1980). Economy in drug prescribing in Mozambique. *Trop. Doc.* **10**, 42-5.
—— Traditional medicine in Mozambique. *Africa Today* (forthcoming).
Bhore Committee (1946). *Report of the health services and development committee.* Government of India, New Delhi.
Choudhury, M. R. (1981). Bangladesh: Planning for health. *Wld Hlth Forum* **2**, 167-73.
Cox, P. (1969). The value of mobile medicine. *E. Afr. med. J.* **46**, 1-5.
Creese, A. (1979). Expanded programme on immunisation: costing guidelines. EPI/GEN/79/5. World Health Organization, Geneva.
Djukanovic, V. and Mach, E. P. (1975). *Alternative approaches to meeting basic health needs in developing countries.* World Health Organization, Geneva.
England, R. (1978). More myths in international health planning. *Am. J. Publ. Hlth* **68**, 153-9.
Fendall, R. (1981). Ayurvedic medicine and primary health care. *Trop. Doc.* **11**, 81-5; reproduced in *Wld Hlth Forum*, **3**, 90-4. (1982).
Gish, O. (1975). *Planning the health sector: the Tanzanian experience.* Croom Helm, London.
—— and Walker, G. (1977). *Mobile health services: a study in cost-effectiveness.* Tri-Med Books, London.
Jagdish, V. (1981). Primary health care in rural India. *Wld Hlth Forum* **2**, 218-21.

Kaprio, L. A. (1979). *Primary health care in Europe.* Euro Report No. 14. World Health Organization, Copenhagen.

Lee, K. (1979). Need versus demand: the planner's dilemma. In *Economics and health planning* (ed. K. Lee) pp. 45–69. Croom Helm, London.

— (1982). Public expenditure, health services and health. In *Public expenditure and social policy* (ed. A. Walker), pp. 73–90. Heinemann, London.

— and Mills, A. (1982). *Policy-making and planning in the health sector.* Croom Helm, London.

Ramalingaswami, V. (ed.) (1981). *Health for all: an alternative strategy.* Indian Council of Medical Research, Indian Institute of Education, Pune.

Ruby, G., Vpahurch, O., and Weisfeld, N. (1977). A manpower policy for primary health care: definition of primary care. Institute of Medicine, Department of Health Manpower, Research and Development, Washington D.C.

Sidel, R. and Sidel, V. W. (1980). China's health care facilities. In *China* (ed. A. J. Keizer and F. M. Kaplan). Eurasia Press, New York.

— (1977). Primary health care in relation to socio-political structure. *Soc. Sci. Med.* 11, 415-19.

Skeet, M. and Elliott, K. (ed.) (1978) *Health auxiliaries and the health team.* Croom Helm, London.

Smith, R. A. (1982). Primary health care—rhetoric or reality? *Wld Hlth Forum* 3, 30-7.

Sorkin, A. L. (1976). *Health economics in developing countries.* D. C. Heath and Co., Massachusetts.

Taylor C. E. (1980). Evaluation methodology in primary health care. National Conference on Evaluation of Primary Health Care Programmes, Indian Council of Medical Research, New Delhi, 21-23 April.

— *et al.* (1976). *Functional analysis of health needs and services.* Asia Publishing House, New Delhi.

Tejada-de-Rivero, D. (1981). W. K. Kellogg Foundation Lecture, First International Course on Education for Health Services' Administration, Lisbon.

Vuori, H. (1982). The World Health Organization and Traditional Medicine. *Community Med.* 4, 129-37.

Walt, G. and Vaughan, P. (1981). *An introduction to the primary care approach in developing countries.* Ross Institute Publications No. 13, London.

WHO (World Health Organization) (1978*a*). *Primary health care.* World Health Organization, Geneva.

— (1978*b*). Financing of health services. *Tech. Rep. Ser. Wld Hlth Org.* **625.**

— (1979). *Formulating strategies for health for all by the year 2000.* World Health Organization, Geneva.

— (1980). Sixth report on the world health situation, 1973-1977. Part I: *Global Analysis.* World Health Organization, Geneva.

— /IND (1980). Strategies for health for all by the year 2000: India. Document SEA/HFA/New Delhi, June.

—/SEARO (1980). *Report of regional meeting on appropriate technology for health in relation to primary health care.* World Health Organization, New Delhi.

— /UNICEF (1980). *Report of interregional workshop on cost and financing patterns of primary health care.* World Health Organization, Geneva.

World Bank (1981). *World development report 1981.* Oxford University Press, New York.

Author's note

The author is especially indebted to the National Institute for Health and Family Welfare, Government of India, New Delhi, for providing the impetus to explore many of the ideas now contained in this chapter. Its staff gave generously of their time and thought to discuss the role of economic analysis in primary health care. Special thanks are due to colleagues at the Nuffield Centre for Health Services Studies, in particular to Carol Barker, Peter Cox, and Jack Hallas, for their comments and advice on an earlier draft of this chapter. None of these persons has seen the final version and can therefore safely be absolved from any errors that remain.

6

Some health manpower policy issues

Geoffrey Ferster and Robert Tilden

National human resource development

A nation's development process is conditioned by its culture, climate, and institutional background as well as by its natural resource base and, in most instances, by conditions that exist outside its borders. Nations consciously striving towards national development do so on the basis of stated goals and principles that the component parts of the socioeconomic development process must reflect. The health sector operates within the bounds of these principles and governments attempt to ensure that all efforts of the government machinery, community, and private sector are directed to these national objectives and strategies.

A major issue in the process of development for many of the developing countries is how to elicit the goodwill and sustained spirit and effort of their people, including their civil servants, the community, and the private sector, to work towards national goals and objectives. Human resource development can thus be seen as a major focal point for any developing country. Hence a nation's policies on manpower become a crucial component in its development process.

In recent decades it has become clear that among a nation's most important resources essential to the development process are its human resources (Becker 1962). Policies for health manpower form part of overall manpower development, while possessing special features of their own. Strong investment in the infrastructure of education and health can satisfy a number of objectives. It can be seen as a good form of income redistribution in kind, especially if these services are provided free or at subsidized prices to low income families who previously did not have sufficient access to them. It also provides the 'raw material' in the form of students who can be given further education and training in health service and health-related activities. Moreover, investments in education have spill-over effects not only on health manpower development, but also on health status itself. It has been shown that literacy, for instance, is a strong determinant of health status in many developing countries (Grosse 1980). Figure 6.1 shows the relationship between literacy and infant mortality rate in 86 LDCs. These findings obviously have a number of policy implications for human resource development (World Bank 1980).

Clearly, a key to the improvement of health status in LDCs is the education

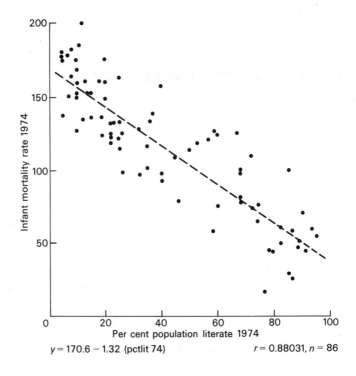

$y = 170.6 - 1.32 \ (\text{pctlit 74})$ $\qquad\qquad$ $r = 0.88031, n = 86$

Fig. 6.1. Literacy and infant mortality rates, 1974.

and training of a range of health workers (both health professionals and non-formal health supporters), and the development of arrangements, techniques, and procedures to ensure their continued productive behaviour. However, little is known about which set of manpower policy approaches might be most appropriate and efficient in addressing the health manpower problems faced by particular countries, and a number of reasons can be advanced for this situation.

First, countries differ in the size, composition, and proportion of public and private resources they devote to health manpower training and skill development. In the public sector in particular, limited resources face competing interests both between and within different manpower groups. Most LDCs, however well intentioned, have been unable to train simultaneously for their country's health services both a limited number of health specialists and a larger amount of middle- and low-level health personnel and trainers. Clearly, policies and action in these areas must influence the quantity and availability of different classes of health manpower.

Secondly, the relationships of inputs to outputs and outcomes in the education process (particularly in the non-formal areas) are not well established and vary among cultures. The field of health is a good example. The well-known uncertainties of the relationship between inputs and outputs for health and medical care are complicated further by the fact that inputs are difficult to quantify, since only a limited proportion of total health care costs are financed by the public sector within developing countries.

Thirdly, the necessary ingredients of motivation, supervision, and support to sustain performance among various levels of health manpower are not well understood. Numerous examples are available to indicate that financial remuneration is an important, though not the sole, determinant for continued high levels of performance and productivity. Further, motivational factors will vary from culture to culture.

Fourthly, health manpower planning needs to be synchronized with other investment policies in human resources to ensure that demand for people with different levels of education are congruent with their supply, and that the plans of one sector are not hampered by those of another.

Fifthly, due to the technical basis of measures required to effect improvements in health, and since knowledge and technology in these areas are in a constant state of change, mechanisms are needed to absorb changing technology and to upgrade health professionals at timely and regular intervals. However, whilst the need for a continuous process for upgrading skills and knowledge is often recognized, uncertainties do exist as to which types of retraining method actually lead to demonstrable cost-effective results. An associated point is that, with the rapid growth in the health services of many LDCs, health professionals are often employed in supervisory roles for which their initial training has not provided the necessary managerial and planning skills. Hence, an ongoing in-service training programme is often needed, particularly to assist health professionals to communicate with specialists in related disciplines, such as management and economics, who can help to improve implementation, evaluation, and supervision at field level.

Sixthly, given the concentration in many LDCs on curative hospital medicine, shortages presently exist of resources and facilities for training the different levels of health professionals in disease prevention and health promotion activities. A set of policies to ensure efficient and effective production of different manpower grades for community health work still needs to be formulated and implemented. For instance, one area where policy-makers are increasingly concentrating their attention is on the training, education, and support of those members of the community who will assist with selected aspects of health development at village level.

Finally, it can be noted that as a nation's health status and human resource development is influenced by a wide set of inputs from sectors outside the health sector, channels of communication on policy issues between these different sectors, and day-to-day communication about management matters between different professional groups, still need to be developed at both the centre and field level to ensure improved implementation of health-related programmes.

Health manpower policy development

Health policy is a statement of intent which seeks to guide sets of inputs (both public and private), organized in particular ways, through a process which leads

to a desired set of outcomes or goals. Policy-making is often exceedingly complicated because of the need to take account of many interdependencies and to
mobilize the necessary resources at all levels. As such, it may not be well understood by the people responsible for carrying it out. Sets of different sector
policies are often also interrelated and this leads to an even greater complexity
in implementation.

In consequence, it is not always entirely obvious how broad national manpower development policies are conceived. Different models have been formulated both to describe and predict policy-making and planning processes (Lee
and Mills 1982). One such model is the advocate (or incremental) model which
suggests that policies tend to emerge as products of conflict from the assertion
of special interests, resulting in various compromises. Such conflict usually takes
place not only in the context of broad national manpower and operational
policies, but also in their translation into annual recruitment and training
strategies. There are clearly both advantages and disadvantages in formulating
components of policies in this manner.

The main advantage in viewing manpower policy-making in this light is that
the involvement of special interests should ensure that they are motivated to
accomplish the goals agreed on (Lindblom 1959). This approach also recognizes
explicitly that local constraints to implementation exist, that divergent views
will persist, and that interested parties need to be made to work together. By
so doing, policy-makers may ensure that finance from both private and public
sources is made available to tackle the necessary problems. The oft-cited dis-
advantage of this approach is that there is often no guarantee that the manpower
requirements for the most important social welfare and health problems will be
effectively met. Hence, the main effort will not necessarily be directed to greater
equity in manpower distribution (spatially or otherwise), and it might or might
not in practice lead to even improved manpower quality. Yet it is often argued
that one of the major justifications for setting health as a goal of development,
and especially for investing public resources in the health sector, is the implied
income transfer and the effects on income distribution (Chenery, Ahluwalia,
Bell, Duloy, and Jolly 1974; Haveman and Weisbrod 1977; Nath 1980).

A second model of decision-making has thus been formulated, entitled the
rational (or comprehensive) approach to manpower policy formulation and
planning. The main value of this model is argued to be that it provides a stepwise
approach to managing the limited resources available for manpower development, albeit in reality the situation is usually more complex (Smith 1976; Hall
and Mejia 1978; Hornby, Ray, Shipp, and Hall 1980). Not only do many unfore-
seen problems arise during the development process, but institutional problems
of inter- as well as intra-sectoral co-ordination can destroy or render ineffective
the best conceived comprehensive manpower plan.

In the context of LDCs, the lack of essential information from national or
field level usually precludes reliance on this type of model, though it may be
useful in giving guidance on what essential information is required to use this

approach in subsequent iterations (Grosse *et al.* 1979). Because these issues of information and related uncertainties are so real, models of 'mixed scanning' have been advocated, whereby manpower models focus selectively upon what essential information is needed in subsequent iterations, and manpower planners focus only on a limited range of feasible alternative plans (Etzioni 1967). Yet the argument in favour of 'rationalism' in manpower planning is that at the very least it does help the manpower policy-maker understand the essential inter-relationships, important trade-offs, and the most significant information gaps. As such, the undertaking of this approach can lead to better policy formulation, regardless of whether or not the information generated is fully used in making the final decisons.

Closely allied to these alternative models of decision-making are issues of decentralization, community participation, and implementation. For instance, one area in national manpower policy that has recently received considerable attention in LDCs is that of decentralization. There are many issues, however, to be resolved within this area, including those of levels of decision-making, financing, and implementation and monitoring. While such a broad spectrum of issues warns against over-generalization on the advantages of decentralization, arguments are advanced that, in order to relate the aims of health manpower development more closely to the needs of the population being served, this complicated process would run more effectively and more efficiently if it were operated at local levels. There are, however, solid reasons why careful phasing of decentralization should take place in most developing countries, thereby causing local areas to be guided from a centralized approach. Apart from the obvious requirements to consider certain manpower issues on a national rather than a regional or district basis, which would be beyond the scope of local organizations, some baseline work at national level may be necessary to determine the parameters within which the local groups can operate. Indeed, to help facilitate a meaningful decentralization, a tremendous reservoir of technically trained manpower is required to take responsibility for handling the complexities of the many programmes. In consequence, whereas decentralization is a valuable goal, the lack of a sufficient number of trained staff will often inhibit progress and cause credibility problems among the population who may have expected superior results in their local areas. Such antipathy must be viewed carefully as it could reduce the goodwill essential for all development efforts to succeed.

A complementary issue to decentralization, and one which is becoming dominant among LDCs, is that associated with the extent of community participation in activities for socioeconomic development. It is clear that not all communities can wait for national manpower plans to come to fruition, or for trained manpower to be available to assist in village level development. Further, it is recognized that some activities are within the scope of community action and could be more efficiently and effectively conducted at the community level. While there are numerous problems associated with community participation, such as how to integrate inter-sectoral projects, provide adequate finance and supervision, and phase community participation within the country, encourageing results from experiments within different sectors at the community level are now being brought to the attention of planners and national leaders, programmes are being assessed and different ways explored to use low-cost human resources in ongoing programmes and to develop primary health care (WHO 1978, 1979; Golladay and Liese 1980; Werner 1981). The health sector has provided examples in several countries. Some of them can be replicated and have been used in some countries as the catalyst for developing multi-sectoral activities in the field (Selowsky 1978; Bairagi 1980). Relevant training, sustained supervision, and adequate support services have been seen in the health sector to be critical parameters in determining the success of PHC projects (WHO 1979).

As regards the implemenation of health manpower policies, most of those experienced in working in developing countries are aware that, even in the most optimistic scenario, improvements in quality of life, economic parameters, and health manpower will not emerge rapidly. At best, progress will follow a gradual incremental path. Three major constraints are apparent. First, judging from the past, abundant resources will not become available for key development areas, even though some countries possibly could make use of a massive infusion of foreign assistance on favourable terms. Even with these resources, the problems of absorption and implementation of health care and basic health promotion activities will remain. Secondly, given the lack of available resources such as manpower, facilities, and finance, hard choices must be made in order to achieve at field level a 'phased-in' set of viable interventions specified to reach target populations at targeted levels. Thirdly, no major dramatic shifts away from a combination of low and high technology programmes in the health sector can be expected. Modification in the resource mix over a period of time would still mean a sizeable proportion of resources would be devoted to the curative aspects of medical care, which it is hoped would include an effective referral system. For example, to illustrate from a related sector, it is hard to imagine that a country would completely abandon all resources for higher education in favour of a broadly based primary school programme, mixed with informal adult education and literacy programmes and middle-level technical training. On the other hand, a programme that stressed only the development of universities would not greatly benefit the common person either.

Developing health manpower

The definitions of health and disease adopted by a mother from a rural area may well be quite different from those of a Western-trained health bureaucrat (Morley 1973). In some countries, this means that community health centres remain underutilized, while traditional medical services apparently do a good business. Often mothers in the villages will try self-medication as an appropriate alternative. An important question, therefore, in manpower planning activity, is how far to take into account the self-perceived needs of the population and, likewise, how far to attempt to educate the population to interact in a positive manner with important health improvement programmes. For instance, one can view the market demand for health as an expression of the communities' health problem priorities or, more precisely, an expression based upon the existing distribution of income and wealth. Quite often this expression will not coincide with the health priorities either as established by the planner or as presently supported. Yet unless some accommodation of needs is made, for instance by altering demand through (say) health education while simultaneously responding to the population's own perceived demands, little can be accomplished (King 1975).

At the same time, with regard to the recruitment and remuneration of health manpower, public policy in many LDCs appears to have been consciously interventionist, aiming to override or affect free labour market forces, especially for skilled manpower, and to depress remuneration levels. A number of reasons can be advanced: first, to ensure that the salaries of health personnel do not engulf all public resources; second, to ensure that the level of remuneration for trained staff is not seen as being wholly out of line with the population they are serving; third, to establish some comparable level of compensation and parity of remuneration for trained staff working at various levels in the public sector.

This role of state employment does become a delicate matter in some LDCs, where part of the health manpower is able to generate private income. Doctors often can, in addition to their public responsibilities, devote some time to establishing private practices: indeed this may be necessary to secure a sufficiently high income to support the expected standard of living. In such countries, a combination of market forces and professional interests can usually be counted upon to produce more or less sizeable income distortions between geographical areas. This is particularly evident between rural and urban areas where the higher urban wage rate for health professionals, arising from greater scope for private practice, appears to have been a major determinant of present geographical inequalities in the distribution of health professionals in many countries. This is an issue that affects more than the medical profession, for the health sector employs a number of workers whose skills are in demand in other industries. Public sector wages must necessarily take note of this fact. By way of an example, many developing countries are in the process of developing computer facilities. Quite often the turnover rate of trained government computer personnel is quite high, as private industry is also looking for the same skills and willing to pay more than the health department. Similar examples can be quoted for trained nurses absorbed into the private sector or into tourist hotels. Indeed, the establishment of village volunteers has often had serious problems due to a high attrition rate. Village volunteers are often expected to serve at little or no pay; this can lead to under-motivation and loss of interest.

To help compensate for the intentionally low salary structure, many health departments have resorted to non-cash benefits, supplying, for instance, free health care, foodstuffs, transportation, housing, and education for children.

While a portion of 'basic needs' can compensate for low salaries, these benefits are sometimes available only for those of the upper echelon, reflecting the greater influence (leverage) that higher level personnel can wield. The lower the pay scales, the more important will be non-cash benefits, or the promise of being able to be promoted in the hierarchical structure, be it in administration or at field level. This incentive may be very important to health manpower with special training; upward mobility can help with motivation and also reduce attrition of all levels of staff.

A good deal has been said about the so-called 'brain drain' (Mejia, Pizurki, and Royston 1979). The negative effects of this in drawing away highly qualified personnel have been well documented. Doctors who emigrate to a Western country are indeed doing both their countries and eventually themselves a disservice, excepting of course that some international jobs with health agencies are best undertaken by administrators familiar with the problems of developing countries. In respect of all sections of health manpower, including doctors, it is abundantly clear that appropriate techniques to maintain motivation of personnel and control systems are crucial, and that salary levels, non-cash benefits, and job satisfaction are all essential ingredients in turning appropriate health manpower planning into effective health programmes.

Health policy and health manpower

A main theme of this chapter so far has been that there are as many important inputs into health manpower development policy as there are into determining a national development policy. One may develop a well-designed 'rational' model for manpower policy that may not meet either the demands of consumers or match the changing disease profile as defined by local and international medical personnel. Likewise, the 'advocate' approach toward manpower planning will probably only deliver those services that the most influential consumers and/or providers demand, and the special interests of different groups, including key political figures, encourage. This approach would thus probably not direct manpower into the roles most effective in reducing excessive mortality and debility, and increasing life expectancy.

Manpower policy should be both a key element of overall development strategy, and reflect other sectors' activities that affect health status, such as agriculture, industry, social welfare, education, and urban planning. It follows that health manpower policy cannot be established separately from health care policy. The basic steps of manpower policy should reflect interaction between all health programmes in the establishment of both short-range and long-term strategies. Only within this framework can a systematic and internally consistent approach to manpower planning be effective. The first few steps of such an approach would involve several aspects relevant to health manpower determination, and might well include the following:

(1) information on health problems, both as defined by a perceived market demand, and as defined epidemiologically;

(2) information and bounded predictions of what the nature and scope of the main health problems will be in both the medium- and longer-term; and
(3) the definition of different types of health programmes, both those in existence and those deemed to be essential in the future. It is hoped that one might also have information about the cost of programme expansion, the impact of these programmes on health, and the resource implications and consequences—including classes of manpower required—of various combinations of the programmes.

Before initiating a thorough analysis of what might be a reasonable set of alternative programmes, and what the medium- and long-range coverage targets are, criteria must be chosen to evaluate the programmes. Ideally, one might try using the cost-effectiveness approach for instance, as pioneered by Grosse *et al.* (1979). However, even if the analysis were to be somewhat less rigorous than this model, some criteria are still required to help explore what alternative mixes of programmes are preferred both in the medium- and longer-term (Walsh and Warren 1979).

A first consideration in comparing alternative programme mixes and their phasing over time is that of resource constraints, including those associated with manpower. One will undoubtedly find that however carefully plans for action for manpower are developed, shortages of some manpower classes will emerge. Hence, the responsibility of government is to try to ensure that those classes and categories which will be needed are trained and upgraded. Further, those who are displaced from work due to, for instance, changes in technologies and the changing demands for some health services should be given a chance to be retrained. But some categories take a long time to educate and train, while others can be trained very quickly. Hence, some priority must be set and personnel trained before they are needed. Using a master plan/PERT (Fulop and Reinke 1981) approach one can perhaps begin to make sure the right amount of the right personnel are available when needed.

A second consideration is that of the degree of occupational and professional mobility within the organization, both in terms of upward mobility (i.e. different levels of seniority in specialized jobs) as well as horizontal mobility (for instance there should be scope for malaria spray workers to be redeployed once malaria is under control, and smallpox vaccinators to be retrained and absorbed in the new programmes of expanded immunization). A further important point is the need for managerial and supervisory staff. At present, quite often there is a tendency to train and deploy new types of field workers with inadequate supervision and lack of infrastructure support.

Related to the above points is a third and important consideration, namely the desirability of creating an inventory of existing health manpower deployed in both the private and public sectors, together with some appreciation of their performance and productivity, and their geographical distribution. From such an inventory, it should become obvious where the deficits in manpower classes would arise in any proposed programme or plan. It should then also be possible to know what the production rates and availability of health manpower could be within both the private and public sectors. It could be very true that the need in certain categories will outstrip the production potential of that category. While an intensive programme for building and training facilities might solve the problem in the short run, in the longer run it may create a glut of health personnel. Deploying out-of-country technicians or international volunteers would be one short-term remedy, though consultants and volunteers, of course, also impose local costs.

Throughout the training and development of health manpower, it is important to monitor their professional development. This will also help in the evaluation of the training curriculum. Two important issues emerge at this point; one concerns maintaining high levels of health manpower motivation, the other is the need to keep up in-service training of health manpower. It is well recognized that the factors involved in motivation are complex and sometimes culturally specific; however, some of the common factors seem to be financial reward, a sense of accomplishment, prestige, an ability to move within the organization both vertically and horizontally, and a feeling that one is a member of a team. All persons would not be expected to place the same level of importance on the same factors; hence, health manpower policy should reflect and be able to adapt to the diverse personal needs of those health workers responsible for the implementation of health policy. Finally, it is essential that programmes be evaluated, both in terms of satisfying current policies as well as in the light of emerging health care needs. This review may lead to redeployment of manpower in certain activities, but is also likely to identify the levels and extent for appropriate in-service training.

Conclusion

This chapter has not attempted to develop a new theory of health manpower development, nor has it tried to offer a 'cook book' set of considerations on how to establish health manpower policy. Instead, what the chapter has tried to address are a number of issues considered to be important in establishing health manpower policy in the developing world.

The main lessons that have emerged include the following:

(1) health manpower development policy cannot be established independently of health care policy in general;

(2) health care policy should be part of a larger concern, that of national development policy;

(3) sectors other than health are often responsible for improvements in health status and, hence, health manpower policy should reflect these cross-linkages;

(4) health manpower policy should reflect also the private sector's manpower demands and availability, and the perceived market demand for health services;

(5) supervision and infrastructure development are essential components of health manpower policy consideration; and finally,

(6) motivational factors of health manpower personnel (including those of community health workers) are essential ingredients in policy considerations.

REFERENCES

Bairagi, R. (1980). Is income the only constraint on child nutrition in rural Bangladesh? *Bull. Wld Hlth Org.* **58**, 767-72.

Becker, G. S. (1962). Investment in human capital: a theoretical analysis. *J. Polit. Econ.* **70**, 9-49.

Chenery, H., Ahluwalia, M. S., Bell, C. C. G., Duloy, J. H., and Jolly, R. (1974). *Redistribution with growth*. Published for the World Bank and Institute of Development Studies, University of Sussex. Oxford University Press.

Etzioni, A. (1967). Mixed scanning: a third approach to decision-making. *Publ. Admin. Rev.* **27**, 385-9.

Fulop, T. and Reinke, W. A. (1981). Statistical analysis of independence of country health resource variables, with special regards to manpower-related ones. *Bull. Wld Hlth Org.* **59**, 129-41.

Golladay, F. and Liese, B. (1980). *Health problems and policies in the developing countries*. Staff Working Paper No. 412. World Bank, Washington DC.

Grosse, R. N. *et al.* (1979). A health development model application to rural Java: draft. Department of Health Planning and Administration, School of Public Health, The University of Michigan, Ann Arbor, Michigan.

— (1980). Interrelationship between health and population: observations derived from field experiences. *Social Sci. Med.* **14C**, 99-120.

Hall, T. L. and Mejia, A. (ed.) (1978). *Health manpower planning*. World Health Organization, Geneva.

Haveman, R. H. and Weisbrod, B. A. (1977). Economic principles for policy analysis. Part Two. In *Public expenditure and policy analysis* (ed. R. H. Haveman and J. Margolis). Rand McNally College Publishing Company, Chicago.

Hornby, P., Ray, D. K., Shipp, P. J., and Hall, T. L. (1980). *Guidelines for health manpower planning*. World Health Organization, Geneva.

King, M. (1975). *Medical care in developing countries*. Oxford University Press, Nairobi.

Lee, K. and Mills, A. (1982). *Policy-making and planning in the health sector*. Croom Helm, London.

Lindblom, C. E. (1959). The science of muddling through. *Publ. Admin. Rev.* **19**, 79-88.

Mejia, A., Pizurki, H., and Royston, E. (1979). *Physician and nurse migration: analysis and policy implications*. World Health Organization, Geneva.

Morley, D. (1973). *Paediatric priorities in developing countries*. Butterworth, London.

Nath, S. K. (1980). *A reappraisal of welfare economics*. Routledge and Kegan Paul, London.

Selowsky, M. (1978). *The economic dimensions of malnutrition in young children: a survey of the issues*. Staff Working Paper No. 294. World Bank, Washington DC.

Smith, A. R. (ed.) (1976). *Some statistical techniques in manpower planning*. Civil Service College Occasional Paper No. 15. HMSO, London.

Walsh, J. A. and Warren, K. S. (1979). Selective primary health care: an interim strategy for disease control in developing countries. *New Engl. J. Med.* **301**, 967–73.

Werner, D. (1981). The village health worker: lackey or liberator? *Wld Hlth Forum* **2**, 46–54.

World Bank (1980). *World Development Report 1980.* World Bank, Washington DC.

WHO (World Health Organization) (1978). *Primary health care: report of the international conference on primary health care*, Alma-Ata. World Health Organization, Geneva.

—— (1979). *Formulating strategies for health for all by the year 2000.* World Health Organization, Geneva.

7

Economic appraisal in the health sector

Nicholas Prescott and Jeremy Warford

Introduction

This paper discusses the role of economic appraisal in the formulation of health
sector policy in less developed countries (LDCs). Specifically, it focuses on the
application of economic analysis to public investment decisions in the health
sector, that is to the design, selection, and financing of projects which constitute
the health component of a development plan. The underlying theme is the
desirability of integrating the health sector more closely with the overall framework of development planning through a systematic process of project appraisal
based on clearly specified objectives and resource constraints.

Generalizations about LDCs as a group are inevitably heroic when—as
defined by the World Bank—they comprise countries as diverse as India,
Lesotho, Fiji, Korea, Brazil, and Chad. However, by definition, all of these
countries share the characteristic of a relatively low level of per capita income
(World Bank 1981), typically associated with a limited tax base due to weak
tax administration and low ratios of taxable surplus to GNP (Tait, Gratz, and
Eichengreen 1979; Meerman 1980). The combination of these factors produces
an acute shortage of resources to finance public expenditure, thus emphasizing
the importance of achieving efficient investment planning in the public sector.
This is particularly true today when the prospects for per capita income growth
in LDCs have deteriorated markedly (World Bank 1981) and the adoption of
structural adjustment policies is enforcing a more rigorous review of public
investment programmes (Balassa 1982). Other characteristics commonly observed
in LDCs include overvalued exchange rates, substantial unemployment or
underemployment, and a skewed income distribution, together with a variety
of constraints which limit the ability of their governments to increase private
savings and redistribute income with the conventional instruments of fiscal
and monetary policy.

These factors have important implications for project selection in the health
sector. Resource allocation decisions have in the past been notoriously inefficient and inequitable, and are now reflected in an emphasis on expensive
urban and hospital-based curative care which is not directed at the major causes
of ill-health in the majority of LDC populations. Moreover, health has tended
to claim a low and often declining share of public expenditure (IMF 1981),
and the prospects for a substantial increase in real budgetary allocations to

the sector are poor. At the same time, recent interest in basic needs and the efforts by WHO and UNICEF to promote 'Health for all by the year 2000' have created ambitious objectives for health improvement in LDCs. The Director-General of WHO has suggested that an infant mortality rate of less than 50 per thousand live births, and a life expectancy at birth greater than 60 years, should be minimum objectives for health improvement by the year 2000 (Mahler 1977). These contrast with infant mortality rates higher than 200 per thousand, and life expectancy lower than 40 years, observed in some low-income LDCs. The financial implications of these objectives are enormous. A recent WHO estimate implies that their achievement would require up to an eightfold increase over the present level of public expenditure on health in low-income LDCs of approximately $2.5 per capita (WHO 1981). However, the health sector continues to operate, to an extent that is unmatched in any other sector, without the guidance of systematic project appraisal criteria which could help to reconcile these health objectives with other development objectives in the face of increasingly severe resource constraints.

It is, therefore, essential to develop ways of improving the efficiency of public expenditure on health in LDCs, and also of mobilizing additional revenue to finance increased levels of expenditure. This chapter examines these issues in the following framework. First, the basic elements of financial analysis which provide the starting point for analysis of efficiency and resource mobilization are discussed. Then there are two sections which review alternative forms of efficiency criteria, namely cost-effectiveness and cost–benefit analysis, with special attention to the treatment of uncertainty and shadow pricing in health projects. The final section concludes with a consideration of cost recovery options to mobilize additional resources from outside the public sector.

Financial analysis

Health ministries, using conventional public accounting procedures in LDCs, are generally unaware in detail of the allocation of public resources between different interventions and its relationship to stated health objectives, or of the unit costs of different interventions, or of the full potential of available sources of finance. The situation is complicated by the activities of numerous other agencies, both public and private, that affect health, major examples being those agencies concerned with water supply, nutrition, and pharmaceutical production and distribution. This lack of basic financial data severely limits the ability of health ministries to make systematic judgements about the merits of existing and proposed expenditure patterns and financing policies in the public sector, and reform of their financial accounting systems is clearly indicated. The starting point for economic analysis of investment decisions should be a detailed analysis of total public and private health-related expenditures in terms of expenditure patterns and sources of finance. Chapter 3 is devoted to this set of issues, but it is appropriate here to highlight a few of the main features.

Expenditure patterns. Analysis of the allocation of public expenditure between different interventions indicates the extent to which the current expenditure pattern responds to a country's major health problems and proclaimed objectives. Thus, it helps to signal the desirability of reallocating existing expenditures or undertaking new investments. If, as rhetoric suggests, distributional objectives are also important, analysis of the distribution of expenditure by beneficiaries in different income classes (Meerman 1979; Selowsky 1979; Tan 1975), or simply by region (Ofosu-Amaah 1975), will be similarly revealing.

Estimates of the unit costs of different interventions, making an appropriate —if not scientific—allocation of joint costs, provide additional signals. Ideally, these should be estimated in terms of long-run marginal costs, which relate capital expansion and recurrent (i.e. operating and replacement) costs to the volume of additional services provided (Saunders, Warford, and Mann 1977). Differences in the unit cost of interventions suggest the possibility of efficiency gains by switching expenditure to lower cost interventions if these are equally effective. The same applies to unit cost differences for similar interventions delivered by different facilities. For example, a study in Malaysia found that the unit cost of out-patient services in rural clinics exceeded those provided by hospitals, suggesting the existence of significant excess capacity in the rural clinic system (Meerman 1979). Similar comparisons can be made between the public and private sectors. Data collected in Lesotho (Smith 1980) indicate that the public sector is a relatively inefficient producer of health services. The average cost per in-patient was almost three times higher in public than private hospitals, and similar differentials existed for hospital and clinic out-patients. Although unadjusted for case-mix and labour cost differences, it is improbable that these factors fully accounted for such high unit cost differentials. Finally, with the objective of cost containment in mind, trends in the unit costs of similar interventions at different points in time may be used to monitor efficiency in service provision.

Sources of finance. In a similar way, analysis of the sources of finance of existing health expenditure patterns—by public revenues, external donors, private consumers, employers, and charity organizations—can provide important signals to more efficient methods of mobilizing resources for the health sector. For example, available data showing that a major proportion of total health expenditure is financed by private consumers (WHO 1977) suggests the existence of a high level of private willingness (and ability) to pay for health services which remains largely untapped by the public sector. This type of analysis relates intimately to the analysis of expenditure patterns since the potential role of various financing mechanisms, ranging from direct user charges at one extreme to full subsidy from public revenues at the other, tends to vary across different interventions.

Recurrent cost financing. A critically important aspect of the analysis of health sector financing, and one which emphasizes the importance of developing alternative cost recovery mechanisms, concerns the future availability of fiscal resources to subsidize the recurrent costs generated by new investment projects in the health sector. The availability of public funds to subsidize ongoing operating and maintenance costs is typically the binding constraint on health investments. The reason is that external finance from aid donors is often forthcoming to cover capital investment costs, while future recurrent costs have to be financed from domestic revenues after project implementation.

The problem of recurrent cost financing for social sector projects was recognized a long time ago (Stolper 1966), and has recently attracted attention throughout the public sector in LDCs (Heller 1979; Club du Sahel 1980). There are a number of reasons why it is especially important in the health sector. First of all, the neglect of project analysis criteria for health projects has tended to preclude attention even to elementary financial appraisal. Secondly, the amount of recurrent expenditure generated per unit of investment in the health sector is typically higher than in most other sectors, principally because of the labour and pharmaceutical requirements of health facilities. Moreover, the amount of recurrent public subsidy paid per unit of recurrent expenditure is also relatively high in the health sector. Most public sector health projects are financed exclusively, or largely so, from public revenues. Health sector pricing policies are such that user charges are frequently nominal and recover only a low proportion of operating costs. In addition, the revenues generated by this or other cost recovery mechanisms usually accrue directly to the central government Treasury, without any earmarked allocation to the health sector or to the project itself. Thus the allocation of investment resources to health tends to have more onerous implications for recurrent expenditure financing than in other sectors.

Public finance constraints have clear implications for the analysis of project choice in the health sector. Whether partially or totally financed by public subsidy, every project requires a cash flow of revenues to cover its financial costs in order to operate at optimal scale. Analysis of expected future financial costs and revenues of the project is critically important to determine the feasibility of a project over its planned operating life. Indeed, analysis of long-run financial feasibility itself provides a partial test of efficiency simply because future underfinancing of recurrent costs will result in the operating of the project at less than optimal scale and, hence, in a reduction in the net benefit of the investment.

A useful way of summarizing the recurrent expenditure implications of health projects is to estimate the ratio of annual recurrent costs to total investment costs, the so-called 'r-coefficient'. For example, $1000 invested in the health sector in Malawi is expected to generate, on average, $250 of incremental recurrent costs per year, compared with only about $100 resulting from the same investment in education or agriculture (World Bank 1982). Moreover, the recurrent cost implications of health investment are higher at lower levels of the health sector. Estimated recurrent cost ratios in Malawi average 0.5 for clinics and primary health care compared to 0.2 for hospitals. Similar patterns have been observed in Kenya and Malaysia (Heller 1974, 1975) and the Sahel countries (Over 1979).

Consideration of financial feasibility leads directly into the analysis of efficiency criteria. Clearly, the objective of planners is not just to ensure a financially feasible choice of health projects but the best choice from various possible alternatives. One approach, using cost–effectiveness analysis, is to select the mix of feasible projects which yields the largest expected improvement in health status, relative to cost. Ideally, the use of cost–benefit analysis would be preferable, to select those projects which have the largest net social benefit, defined in terms of a wider set of development objectives. Some of the key problems involved in cost–effectiveness and cost–benefit analysis are considered below.

Cost–effectiveness analysis

The least controversial efficiency criterion for health project selection, that of cost–effectiveness, is to choose projects which yield the maximum health improvement subject to available resources. Alternatively, the problem can be inverted to choose projects which minimize the cost of meeting a specified objective or objectives.Cost–effectiveness analysis (CEA) is frequently used in sectors where problems of benefit valuation occur. For example, electricity investment planning models are typically specified in cost-minimization form, to find the least-cost solution to meeting an exogenous future demand upon which a value may or may not be placed (Turvey and Anderson 1977). The method lends itself naturally to the health sector where the concept of meeting basic needs suggests that quantifiable minimum standards exist and can serve as planning objectives. Unfortunately, the basic needs literature is still distinguished by an absence of concrete suggestions as to what these standards should be (see, for example, Streeten, Burki, Ul Haq, Hicks, and Stewart 1981, or Richards and Leonor 1982).

A fundamental problem in applying CEA to the health sector lies in the choice of an appropriate unit of effectiveness to measure the output of health projects. It may seem obvious that health improvement is the primary objective of public expenditure on health. Effectiveness measures framed in terms of intermediate or service outputs, such as provision of MCH services, are therefore inadequate tests since they do not measure actual improvements in health status. However, a central difficulty in measuring health status is that it is not homogeneous, since health project outputs comprise reductions in both morbidity and mortality. These two types of health improvement can be measured in different ways or aggregated into a composite measure which can itself be constructed in different ways. Examples of alternative approaches are discussed below.

Morbidity reduction. The most straightforward, but limited, measure of health impact is the reduction in the prevalence or incidence of a specific disease. An example is provided by Rosenfield, Smith, and Wolman (1977), who used a simple model of schistosomiasis transmission to simulate the effectiveness in Iran of different control techniques (mollusciciding, engineering measures, chemotherapy, and a combination of these) subject to a given resource constraint over seven years. Maximum output, specified in terms of the greatest reduction in the prevalence rate obtained by the end of the seven-year period, was achieved with a combination of chemotherapy and mollusciciding. This intervention reduced the prevalence rate from 64 per cent to 20 per cent, whereas the next best alternative, chemotherapy, achieved a terminal prevalence rate of 60 per cent. This measure of effectiveness did not take account of the prevalence reductions achieved during the period. A more appropriate measure, in terms of the total number of cases of schistosomiasis prevented over the period, changed the ranking of alternatives. Chemotherapy yielded the greatest output at a cost per case prevented of $1.26, followed by the combination of controls with a unit cost of $1.29.

Measures of effectiveness specified in terms of cases of a disease prevented tend to limit the application of CEA to the choice between different methods of controlling that disease, and preclude its use to evaluate the choice between interventions directed at different diseases. This is so because different diseases have different effects on the duration and extent of morbidity, and also mortality, which are not captured by measures of cases prevented.

A more useful measure which would permit comparison of the morbidity effects of the prevention of different types of diseases is the number of days of disability prevented. This can be expressed as the number of days on which individuals would have experienced some degree of dysfunction due to the relevant disease, and can be weighted to reflect the degree of impairment. Paqueo (1976) illustrates the use of a weighted measure to show higher morbidity rates below the poverty line in the Philippines. An unweighted measure has been used in Indonesia by Grosse, De Vries, Tilden, Dievler, and Day (1979) and Grosse (1980) in a detailed simulation of the effectiveness of alternative health interventions directed at 31 diseases, and subject to seven alternative resource constraints. The choice of activities comprised 48 possible combinations of curative and preventive interventions based on health centres, health sub-centres and village health workers, and sanitation, immunization, and nutrition programmes. Resource constraints varied from $2.06 to $30.00 per capita per year. Simulations at each level of resource availability identified the mix of interventions which minimized the number of days of incapacitating illness per person per year from all causes. At all resource levels health centres were selected but with varying combinations of other inputs. At $5.00 per capita these included village health workers and an immunization programme; at $15.00 a sanitation programme only; and at $30.00 village health workers together with sanitation, immunization, and nutrition programmes.

Mortality reduction. As is the case with morbidity, mortality reduction can be quantified in different ways. The simplest measure, the number of deaths prevented, has the advantage of not being disease-specific and therefore can be used to compare interventions against different diseases. However, in the aggregation of deaths prevented it implicitly assigns the same weight to all regardless of the age at death, whereas a social premium may be attached to the prevention of, for instance, infant deaths or deaths occurring in the productive age groups. Social preferences of this kind can be introduced by using methods which weight deaths prevented at different ages by the additional years of life accruing to the survivors.

One approach is to assume that all survivors live to some arbitrarily determined age. For example, Romeder and McWhinnie (1977) suggest a measure of potential years of life lost (gained) could be given by taking the difference between age at death and 70 years. Other methods take the terminal year as life expectancy at birth, or the life table age at which fewer than an arbitrary proportion, such as 10 per cent, of the original radix are survivors. These methods are unsatisfactory because they do not take account of the probability of survival from the age at death to the hypothetical terminal year. It is more appropriate to measure the potential years of life gained by the expectation of life at the age at which death is averted, estimated from the relevant life table. Other refinements have also been suggested, particularly to take account of selective biases which cause the survival chances of survivors from some causes of death to differ from the cohort average (Shepard and Zeckhauser 1980), as may be the case with measles vaccination in LDCs (The Kasongo Project Team 1981). Weighting for specific age groups can be made even more extreme by simply giving zero weight to certain age groups. Thus planners may be interested exclusively in minimizing infant and child mortality, or adult mortality. The conventional arguments for population control in LDCs could, of course, imply a very low weight for infant and child mortality reductions (depending on one's view of the child survival hypothesis).

The optimal choice of interventions by mortality-based effectiveness measures tends to be different from that resulting from morbidity criteria. For instance, the Grosse model also simulated the effectiveness of intervention alternatives in reducing mortality. For five of the seven different resource constraints the optimal combination of inputs differed substantially according to the choice of objective. For example at $15.00 per capita, the minimum crude death rate was obtained with a health centre combined with village health workers and nutrition and immunization programmes; this compared to the health centre plus sanitation programme choice which minimized days of illness. Adopting the minimization of infant mortality instead of total mortality as the planning objective apparently altered the choice of interventions by introducing nutrition programmes more frequently into the optimal solutions. A similar analysis using a programming model to determine the optimal mix of activities to minimize infant and child mortality has been carried out by Barnum, Barlow, Fajardo, and Pradilla (1980) with data from Colombia.

Composite measures. Since morbidity and mortality objectives tend to have different implications for the best choice of health interventions, it seems preferable to construct a composite measure of health improvement, that is one which aggregates morbidity and mortality reductions. Attempts to construct a so-called health status index have generated a considerable literature relating to developed countries (Culyer, Lavers, and Williams 1971; Berg 1973), but very little concerning LDCs. The central concept underlying this approach is that at any point in time an individual occupies one of a continuum of possible health states ranging from good health to death. For estimation purposes the continuum is divided into discrete health states, $j = 1 \ldots n$. Each state is assigned a value U_j on a utility scale ranging from 0 to 1. Health interventions alter the probability of occupying different health states. The effectiveness of an intervention is measured in terms of the increment in health status units, defined as the discounted sum over all years of the number of days changed from state j to k in each year, multiplied by the utility weight of state k net of the utility weight of state j (Torrance 1976). Methods which have been used in attempts to derive utility weights on the basis of individual preferences, including the Von Neumann-Morgenstern standard gamble approach, are reviewed in Culyer (1978). Effectiveness measures of this type are sometimes called quality-adjusted life years. An illustration of the application of this approach to measurement of the health benefits of the reduction in schistosomiasis and cholera prevalence attributable to water supply improvement in LDCs is presented in Saunders and Warford (1976).

A variant of the health status index approach has been developed and applied in Ghana by the Ghana Health Assessment Project Team (1981). Prevention of death from a specific cause results in a gain of healthy days of life: this gain is computed as the life expectancy at age at death from that cause, converted to the equivalent in days. Prevention of disability from a given cause yields an increase in healthy days equivalent to the expected duration of disability in days weighted by the degree of disability per day (assigned arbitrarily). The sum of both the mortality and morbidity components then provides a measure of effectiveness in terms of healthy days of life saved. An empirical application of this method of ranking 48 causes of morbidity and mortality in Ghana showed the dominant effect of mortality on the selection of disease priorities.

These experiments with different approaches to cost–effectiveness analysis in LDCs suggest two important observations. First, since the most effective choice of health interventions appears to be quite sensitive to changes in resource constraints, however health objectives are formulated, accurate specification of these constraints is critically important to avoid getting locked into inefficient strategies. As noted previously, an assessment of the future availability of recurrent cost financing is especially critical. Second, because the optimal mix of interventions is also sensitive to the choice of health objectives, it is equally important that these should be clearly articulated. This presents particularly formidable problems in practice. Most health plans formulate health objectives in terms of desired resource inputs or intermediate outputs rather than health improvement targets, in part because the health impact of particular inputs and interventions is often not known with any certainty. Moreover, specification of the trade-off between morbidity and mortality objectives necessarily raises fundamental questions about the relative value of different types of health improvement which policy-makers are notoriously reluctant to confront explicitly, even though such trade-offs are implicit in all resource allocation decisions they make. Yet those value judgements have to be made explicit in order to determine, through CEA, an efficient allocation of resources between the full range of potential interventions.

Cost–benefit analysis

The usefulness of CEA in project selection is strictly limited by its measurement of project outputs in physical units which cannot be compared directly with costs. The fact that a least-cost solution exists to meeting a given health objective says nothing about the desirability of achieving that objective in terms of the relationship between social benefits and costs. Moreover its necessarily limited focus on health benefits alone implies that other objectives are unimportant, whereas policy-makers typically seek to pursue several social objectives of which health improvement is only one. The idea that the social benefits of a health improvement project should be measured in terms of its contribution to different social objectives such as increased per capita income and equity in addition to health improvement is advocated by Feldstein (1970), Paglin (1974) and Barlow (1976, 1980), though a dissenting note is offered by Loucks (1975) who excludes health improvement from a long list of development policy objectives. This section examines in the context of LDCs the distinctive problem which arises in applying the CBA approach to health projects, namely the choice of an appropriate measure of the value of health benefits.

The conventional approach to benefit valuation in project analysis is to rely on individual valuations as revealed by consumer behaviour. In a perfectly competitive economy, consumers' willingness to pay for a project output is equal to the prevailing market price. Thus in many cases project outputs can be valued directly at market prices. However, health projects generally cannot be handled in this way. First, the prevalence of zero or heavily subsidized market prices in the health sector results in an absence of observable market data from which to deduce willingness-to-pay. Secondly, where such data are available they may underestimate the true social benefits of intervention if, because of externalities, the consumer is not the sole beneficiary of the output. Preventive interventions directed at communicable diseases, such as immunizations, present a classic example of where the benefits to society are greater than those which accrue to their immediate consumers. Thirdly, market price data may also be unsatisfactory if consumers are not well informed about the benefit to themselves of health services. This again may be especially true of preventive interventions. Finally, even if acceptable measures of private valuations are available from market data, consumer preferences might be rejected in favour of socially determined consumption patterns, not least because the consumption patterns of individuals will reflect a particular distribution of income and wealth. The notion that health and certain other goods such as nutrition and education merit higher levels of consumption than would normally occur without public intervention underlies the basic needs approach to development planning.

Consideration of these conceptual and empirical difficulties has necessitated resort to indirect methods of valuation. At least five major alternatives have been attempted. The most common method is the *human capital* approach. Health improvement is treated as an investment in human capital formation which yields an incremental flow of future income or output (Grossman 1972). Health improvement exerts both quantity and quality effects on the effective supply of labour. Mortality reduction increases the stock of potential workers and hence the potential flow of labour services. Morbidity reduction increases the potential number or efficiency of the flow of labour services. This increment in labour units over time can be estimated and multiplied by their marginal product in order to provide an estimate of the incremental output attributable to any given health improvement (Mushkin 1962). Classic applications of this method are estimates of the economic cost of disease in the United States by Weisbrod (1961), and Rice (1966). In the context of LDCs, the theme of the output-augmenting effects of disease control has been expanded to include its impact on the effective supply of land (attributable to migration induced by the elimination of disease vectors) and accumulation of the capital stock (resulting from a reallocation of private and public expenditure from consumption to savings and investment). For a general review, see Barlow (1979) and Ram and Schultz (1979).

Application of the human capital approach faces certain empirical difficulties, notably in estimating the increment in effective labour supply resulting from morbidity reduction and the marginal product which should be assigned to it. As it is rather easy to apply compared with other approaches it has been used extensively, although there is widespread dissatisfaction with it on conceptual grounds. The method values health only to the extent that it is an investment good which increases aggregate output; it assigns no value to health as a consumption good. Accordingly, it implies that the value of health is greater for those with higher earnings and therefore discriminates against the young, the aged, females, and the poor.

Two alternatives to the human capital approach reflect a desire to base health benefit valuation on consumer preferences. *Implicit private* valuations have been sought in analyses of revealed market preferences in the United States. Blomquist (1979) derived a value of life equal to $387 000 from an analysis of the use of automobile seat belts which yielded a small reduction in the statistical probability of death. In an analysis of risk-compensating wage differentials in the labour market, Thaler and Rosen (1975) estimated the implicit value of life at $176 000. An alternative approach using questionnaire surveys designed to elicit an *explicit private* valuation of mortality reduction has been applied by Acton (1973) to changes in the risk of cardiovascular mortality. He obtained a value of life ranging between $28 000 and $43 000. For a review of these and other consumer preference models see Linnerooth (1979). This approach has not yet been applied to changes in morbidity, or in an LDC context.

Other approaches attempt to replace individual valuations by social preferences. A number of attempts to elicit *implicit public* values, as revealed by government choices in the United Kingdom, are summarized by Card and Mooney (1977). The range of implicit values placed on human life by various programmes or regulations were as follows: £50 in screening maternal oestriol concentration to prevent stillbirths; £1000 in the provision of child-proof drug containers; £100 000 in legislation on tractor cabs; £20 000 000 in building regulations for high-rise apartment blocks. The extreme inconsistency revealed in implicit values across these different public policy areas clearly suggests that this approach serves more as an indicator of the undesirable consequences of *ad hoc* decision-making rather than as a reliable guide to valuing benefits. Feldstein (1970) has suggested instead that *explicit public* values could be obtained by direct questioning of public policy-makers. This idea is similar to the general procedure proposed by Dasgupta, Marglin, and Sen (1972) for the derivation of social weights in project appraisal. A variation of this approach, involving social specification of a basic needs standard for calorie consumption, has been developed by Scandizzo and Knudsen (1980).

The health economics literature offers many examples of cost–benefit analysis (Culyer, Wiseman, and Walker 1977; Griffiths, Rigoni, Tacier, and Prescott 1980; Drummond 1980*a,b*), but there have been few applications to LDCs. All of these concern communicable disease control projects, mainly immunization programmes (see Chapter 8), or parasitic disease control. Such analyses, especially of parasitic disease control, exemplify many of the empirical difficulties encountered in benefit valuation. For example, various studies have assumed that schistosomiasis entails, on average, an impairment of working efficiency ranging from between 4 per cent to 100 per cent. This upper limit is inconsistent with epidemiological evidence that only a minority of infected cases sustain infections of sufficient intensity to provoke clinically severe morbidity, and corroborative physiological evidence from Sudan that significant reductions in physical performance capacity (up to 20 per cent of maximum aerobic power output) are obtained only at very high levels of infection intensity (2000 eggs/g faeces in *S. Mansoni* infections) (Prescott 1979*a*). Similarly, analyses of malaria control have included assumptions about the duration of disability associated with the acute clinical attack (varying from 6 to 44 days) in excess of that which has been observed empirically (2.4 to 5.7 days depending on the species of parasite and the level of host immunity). Such studies have also generally failed to recognize the zero marginal product of additional labour inputs at seasonal periods of labour surplus (Prescott 1979*b*, 1980). Most fundamentally, these analyses have not made realistic predictions of the epidemiological effectiveness of disease control interventions. Like many estimates of the economic cost of disease in developed countries, they are really abstract measures of the gain that could be attributed to hypothetical elimination of a given disease for a single year. Thus they have not addressed the policy-relevant question of what benefits could be generated over time with the application of feasible control techniques.

It is clear that the issue of benefit valuation in health projects has not been resolved satisfactorily, and no single 'correct' method exists which can be recommended to project analysts in LDCs. All of the approaches reviewed have some merits and the choice of a benefit measure will vary in different circumstances. At a minimum, efforts should be made to estimate the unit cost of achieving health improvements with different interventions, so that at least some sensible judgements may be made in the choice between alternative expenditures. Even this needs refinement of basic epidemiological data and analysis, and is but a first step to more powerful analysis involving benefit valuations.

Uncertainty and shadow pricing

The need to take account of uncertainty and to use appropriate 'shadow' prices applies to project analysis, both CEA and CBA, in all sectors but these techniques deserve special mention in the context of health project investment appraisal.

Uncertainty. Uncertainty over the true value of basic parameters in CEA or CBA calculations is inherent in project analysis, partly because by definition the future is unknown and partly because of practical limitations in the quality of relevant data. For instance, a special feature of health projects is the degree of uncertainty about the technology of health improvement. Not enough is known about the relevant production functions, that is the relationship between inputs and outputs, to predict with confidence the health outputs that will result from health project inputs. This fact partly stems from the unusual complexity of health sector production functions. With the exception of preventive interventions which have the characteristic of 'public' goods, improvements in health are produced jointly by health service providers and consumers. Consumer demand is therefore one of the determinants of improved health but knowledge about its characteristics is limited by a lack of empirical data on consumer demand functions for health services and health-related activities.

Another source of uncertainty relates to the technical efficacy of some health interventions in compliant populations, for example BCG vaccination against tuberculosis (Tuberculosis Prevention Trial 1979), or improved water supply and sanitation facilities (World Bank 1975; Saunders and Warford 1976). In addition, uncertainty exists about the accuracy of much of the basic epidemiological data on the incidence or prevalence of morbidity and mortality due to specific causes against which project interventions are directed. For example, estimates of the health benefits of schistosomiasis control are sensitive to assumptions about the morbidity and mortality which it causes, a matter which continues to be the subject of controversy. Apart from such uncertainty about quantifying the benefits of health projects, further uncertainty arises over the value which should be placed on them.

In practice, this problem of uncertainty should be handled by basing the project analysis on best estimates of the basic project parameters, and then analysing the sensitivity of the conclusions to plausible variations of the parameter values around their expected values. The sensitivity analysis will indicate which, if any, of the basic assumptions have a significant effect on the acceptability of a project. The converse approach is to estimate how much different parameter values would have to change before the project switches from being acceptable to unacceptable (or vice versa), and to check whether these are plausible. Such an approach is especially well suited to handling the pervasive uncertainty in health sector projects. Given that in some projects only costs may be known with any confidence, the minimum health output (such as lives saved) required to make the project acceptable can still be estimated and then checked to see whether it is plausible. These estimates can be done within either a CEA or CBA framework.

Shadow pricing. The idea of 'shadow' pricing is to determine the 'real' price of a good or service either where no market price exists or where such a market price is considered to be an incorrect indicator of its 'real' value. In the analysis of health investments, two kinds of shadow prices need to be considered: economic (or efficiency) prices which correct for distortions in factor and product market prices; and social (or distributional) prices which reflect a government's growth and equity objectives. The two main systems of shadow pricing are those developed by Dasgupta *et al.* (1972) and Little and Mirrlees (1974), later refined by Squire and Van der Tak (1975). A full account of the justification for, and derivation of, shadow prices is available in these original sources; only the major points are summarized here.

The use of economic prices mainly affects the value of foreign exchange and labour inputs used by projects. In most LDCs it is common to encounter exchange rates which tend to underestimate the scarcity value of foreign exchange. Conversely, market wage rates often tend to overestimate the opportunity cost of labour. In these circumstances, the effect of the use of 'shadow' prices will be to increase the cost of foreign exchange and reduce the cost of labour. These adjustments will discourage projects which use scarce foreign exchange and favour those which are labour intensive. Likewise, if faster economic growth or income redistribution are key social objectives, then shadow prices in the form of social prices may be used to bias project selection against investment projects which rely heavily on public sector financing, in favour of those which generate high rates of saving and reinvestment by, for example, generating additional public revenue from user charges, and those which redistribute income to the poor.

Some features of the health sector make consideration of shadow pricing of special interest, and the use of economic and social prices has important implications for the choice of health projects. The penalty attached to foreign exchange intensive projects, as a result of the use of economic prices, gives particular importance to pharmaceutical policies directed at minimizing the use of imported pharmaceuticals and increasing domestic production, including primary manufacture which may not rely on imported inputs. The mutually reinforcing incentives to employ labour with a low opportunity cost (for efficiency reasons) and to favour employment of the poor (for distributional reasons) emphasize the desirability of substituting lower for higher grade health workers where technically feasible. The disincentive to using scarce public resources to finance health projects directs attention to exploring methods of self-financing. It is pertinent to observe that all of these concerns—pharmaceutical policy, the use of village health workers and community participation in project financing—are currently the subject of intense policy debate and can each be accommodated through a straightforward application of shadow pricing in project selection.

Resource mobilization

Existing and prospective financial constraints in LDCs indicate a need to re-evaluate the traditional approach to health sector financing which relies heavily on public subsidies from central government revenues. A significant increase in the allocation of public revenues to the health sector is unlikely to be a realistic option, given the traditional strength of competing sectoral demands and the continuing difficulty of demonstrating that the marginal social rate of return on health expenditure exceeds the returns yielded in other sectors. Expansion of the health sector in many countries may, therefore, depend largely on the implementation of cost recovery mechanisms. In general, the relevance of alternative financing methods will vary with the type of health intervention. In each case the choice between financing alternatives can be assessed using the same framework already developed for other public sector projects in which efficiency, equity and fiscal objectives are traded off for the various services provided (Ray 1975).

The benchmark for analysis of financing alternatives is given by the long-run marginal cost of each intervention, though departures from marginal cost pricing can be justified in certain circumstances. In the presence of externalities or poorly informed consumers, both being characteristic of preventive interventions aimed at individuals, marginal cost prices will fail to induce socially optimal levels of consumption, and subsidized prices are appropriate. Public health measures, such as mollusciciding for schistosomiasis control and aerial larviciding for onchocerciasis control, have some of the characteristics of 'public goods', where the benefits of intervention are not consumed by any one individual and the exclusion principle therefore fails to apply, in that access to the benefits of intervention cannot be made conditional on payment of a user charge. Direct charges for such services, levied separately on each beneficiary, may either be too expensive to administer, or simply not feasible.

The achievement of equity objectives will also be affected by the choice of financing mechanism. Interventions directed at low income beneficiaries, for example a programme of primary health care, may be ineffective under a system of direct user charges if the price elasticity of demand is high, meaning that potential consumers are deterred from seeking care by the level of prices charged. Evidence on price elasticities for health services is scarce, but data from Malaysia indicate that the total demand is highly inelastic with respect to cash prices, although there are significant cross-price elasticities for the services of different providers (Heller 1982), implying that consumers do switch between providers according to variations in prices. Similar findings have been reported for the Philippines (Akin, Griffin, Guilkey, and Popkin 1982). If demand is inelastic, the impact of raising charges on the use of health services will by definition be minor and its fiscal impact positive, but the income transfer from the beneficiary to the public sector may not accord with distributional objectives. However, even where these difficulties apply, there may be no alternative but to generate revenues from beneficiaries or elsewhere in the private sector in order to finance the provision of health services.

It is clear, none the less, that for some interventions reliance on direct user charges will not be appropriate and other financing mechanisms will need to be explored. But whether the very limited resort to user charges in LDCs is appropriate—less than 10 per cent of public sector costs are recovered by this means in countries such as Malaysia, Malawi, Lesotho, and Ghana (Brooks 1981)—requires detailed examination. In general, the arguments against pricing are stronger for preventive interventions and for lower income beneficiaries. Thus a system of selective charges for curative services, especially for higher income users, may be justified to cross-subsidize preventive activities and utilization by the poor. Private sector experience, notably of mission facilities and traditional practitioners and birth attendants, demonstrates the feasibility of recovering a high proportion of recurrent costs from user charges without reducing utilization. In Lesotho, some 70 per cent of recurrent expenditure by private hospitals is recovered from user charges (Kolobe and Pekeche 1980).

Alternatives to charges in use in many countries include earmarked taxes, social security and insurance schemes, or indirect cost recovery by self-help (Evans, Hall, and Warford 1981). These methods are explored in Chapters 3 and 4 of this volume, which show that a wide range of financing mechanisms can be employed in the health sector in LDCs. Nevertheless, the approaches generally used are dominated by the tradition of central government subsidy and the introduction of innovative methods encounters very difficult political obstacles. The prevalent view that because health is good it should be free or subsidized may have to be increasingly challenged, however, if the goals set by WHO and UNICEF, referred to in the introduction, are to be achieved.

Conclusion

In general, conventional approaches to investment appraisal in the health sector are much less rigorous than in most other sectors. A major reason for this may be that there are greater difficulties of theory and measurement at all stages of project analysis, for example in the prediction of effectiveness of health interventions, the valuation of benefits, and the design of appropriate cost recovery policies. However, these problems differ in degree rather than substance from those found in other sectors such as water supply, energy, and education, where considerable analytical progress has been achieved. They certainly do not justify the prevalent tendency to avoid rigorous analysis of investment decisions altogether simply because it is difficult. It may even be argued that many of the problems which are encountered are the result of past neglect of economic analysis in the health sector. The potential role of economic appraisal is therefore very large and, indeed, essential to attainment of the dramatic improvements in health status which are now sought by LDCs.

REFERENCES

Acton, J. P. (1973). *Evaluating public programs to save lives: the case of heart attacks*, R-950-RC. The Rand Corporation, Santa Monica, California.
Akin, J. S., Griffin, C. C., Guilkey, D. K., and Popkin, B. M. (1982). The demand for primary health care services in the Bicol region of the Philippines. Paper presented at the National Council for International Health Conference on Financing Health Services in Developing Countries, 14–16 June, Washington DC.
Balassa, B. (1982). Structural adjustment policies in developing economies. *World Development* **10**, 23–38.
Barlow, R. (1976). Applications of a health planning model in Morocco. *Int. J. Hlth Serv.* **6**, 103–21.
— (1979). Health and economic development: a theoretical and empirical review. *Res. hum. Capital Dev.* **1**, 45–75.
— (1980). Economic goals in health planning. Document TDR/SER/SWG(2)/80.WP.6. World Health Organization, Geneva.
Barnum, H., Barlow, R., Fajardo, L., and Pradilla, A. (1980). *A resource allocation model for child survival*. Oelgeschlager, Gunn, and Hain, Cambridge, Mass.
Berg, R. L. (ed.) (1973). *Health status indices*. Hospital Research and Educational Trust, Chicago.
Blomquist, G. (1979). Value of life saving: implications of consumption activity. *J. Polit. Econ.* **87**, 540–58.
Brooks, R. G. (1981). *Ghana's health expenditures 1966–80: a commentary*. Strathclyde Discussion Papers in Economics No. 80/1, University of Strathclyde, Glasgow, Scotland.
Card, W. J. and Mooney, G. H. (1977). What is the monetary value of a human life? *Br. med. J.* **ii**, 1627–9.
Club du Sahel (1980). *Recurrent costs of development programs in the countries of the Sahel: analysis and recommendations*. Club du Sahel, Paris.
Culyer, A. J. (1978). Need, values and health status measurement. In *Economic aspects of health services* (ed. A. J. Culyer and K. G. Wright). Martin Robertson, London.

— Lavers, R. J., and Williams, A. (1971). Social indicators: health. *Soc. Trends* 2, 31–42.
— Wiseman, J., and Walker, A. (1977). *An annotated bibliography of health economics, English language sources.* Martin Robertson, London.
Dasgupta, P. S., Marglin, S. A., and Sen, A. K. (1972). *Guidelines for project evaluation.* United Nations Industrial Development Organization, New York.
Drummond, M. F. (1980a). *Principles of economic appraisal in health care.* Oxford University Press, New York.
— (1980b). *Studies in economic appraisal in health care.* Oxford University Press, New York.
Evans, J. R., Hall, K. L., and Warford, J. J. (1981). Shattuck lecture—Health care in the developing world: problems of scarcity and choice. *New Engl. J. Med.* 305, 1117–27.
Feldstein, M. S. (1970). Health sector planning in developing countries. *Economica* 37, 139–63.
— Piot, M. A., and Sundaresan, T. K. (1973). Resource allocation model for public health planning: a case study of tuberculosis control. *Bull. Wld Hlth Org.* 48, Suppl.
Ghana Health Assessment Project Team (1981). A quantitative method of assessing the health impact of different diseases in less developed countries. *Int. J. Epidemiol.* 10, 73–80.
Griffiths, A., Rigoni, R., Tacier, P., and Prescott, N. (1980). *An annotated bibliography of health economics, Western European sources.* Martin Robertson, Oxford.
Grosse, R. N. (1980). Interrelation between health and population: observations derived from field experiences. *Social Sci. Med.* 14c, 99–120.
— De Vries, J. L., Tilden, R. L., Dievler, A., and Day, S. R. (1979). *A health development model: application to rural Java.* Department of Health Planning and Administration, School of Public Health, The University of Michigan, Ann Arbor, Michigan.
Grossman, M. (1972). On the concept of health capital and the demand for health. *J. Polit. Econ.* 223–55.
Heller, P. S. (1974). Public investment in LDCs with recurrent cost constraints: the Kenyan case. *Q. J. Econ.* 88, 251–77.
— (1975). *Issues in the costing of public sector outputs: the public medical services of Malaysia.* Staff Working Paper No. 207. World Bank, Washington DC.
— (1979). The underfinancing of recurrent development costs. *Finance Dev.* 16, 38–41.
— (1982). A model of the demand for medical and health services in peninsular Malaysia. *Social Sci. Med.* (forthcoming).
IMF (International Monetary Fund) (1981). *Government finance statistics yearbook.* Vol. V, International Monetary Fund, Washington DC.
Kasongo Project Team (1981). Influence of measles vaccination on survival pattern of 7–35 month old children in Kasongo, Zaïre. *Lancet* 764–7.
Kolobe, P. and Pekeche, T. (1980). A survey of the financial status of the private health association of Lesotho's hospitals. Private Health Association of Lesotho, Maseru.
Linnerooth, J. (1979). The value of human life: a review of the models. *Econ. Inquiry* 17, 52–74.
Little, I. M. D. and Mirrlees, J. A. (1974). *Project appraisal and planning for developing countries.* Heinemann Educational Books, London.

Loucks, D. P. (1975). Planning for multiple goals. In *Economy-wide models and development planning* (ed. C. R. Blitzer, P. B. Clark, and L. Taylor), pp. 213–33. Oxford University Press, London.

Mahler, H. (1977). Blueprint for health for all. *WHO Chron.* **31**, 491–8.

Meerman, J. (1979). *Public expenditure in Malaysia: who benefits and why.* Oxford University Press, New York.

— (1980). Paying for human development. In *Implementing programs of human development* (ed. P. T. Knight), pp. 111–82. Staff Working Paper No. 403. World Bank, Washington DC.

Mushkin, J. (1962). Health as an investment. *J. Polit. Econ.* **70**, 129–57.

Ofosu-Amaah, S. (1975). Reflections on the health budget: a preliminary analysis of the 1974/75 Ministry of Health Budget. *Ghana med. J.* 215–22.

Over, A. M. (1979). *Five primary care projects in the Sahel and the issue of recurrent costs.* Harvard Institute for International Development, Cambridge, Massachusetts.

Paglin, M. (1974). Public health and development: a new analytical framework. *Economica* **41**, 432–41.

Paqueo, V. (1976). Social indicators for health and nutrition. In *Measuring Philippine development: report of the social indicators project* (ed. M. Mangahas), pp. 41–115. Development Academy of the Philippines, Manila.

Prescott, N. M. (1979a). Schistosomiasis and development. *Wld Dev.* **7**, 1–14.

—(1979b). The economics of malaria, filariasis and human trypanosomiasis. Document TDR/SER(SC-1)/80.4. World Health Organization, Geneva.

— (1980). On the benefits of tropical disease control. In *Health policies in developing countries* (ed. C. Wood and Y. Rue), pp. 41–8. Royal Society of Medicine International Congress and Symposium Series No. 24. Academic Press, London.

Ram, R. and Schultz, T. W. (1979). Life span, health, savings and productivity. *Econ. Dev. cultural change* **27**, 399–421.

Ray, A. (1975). *Cost recovery policies for public sector projects.* Staff Working Paper No. 206. World Bank, Washington DC.

Rice, D. P. (1966). *Estimating the cost of illness.* Health Economics Series No. 6, PHS Publication No. 947–6. US Government Printing Office, Washington DC.

Richards, P. and Leonor, M. (ed.) (1982). *Target setting for basic needs.* International Labour Office, Geneva.

Romeder, J. M. and McWhinnie, J. R. (1977). Potential years of life lost between ages 1 and 70: an indicator of premature mortality for health planning. *Int. J. Epidemiol.* **6**, 143–51.

Rosenfield, P. L., Smith, R. A., and Wolman, M. G. (1977). Development and verification of a schistosomiasis transmission model. *Am. J. trop. Med. Hyg.* **26**, 505–16.

Saunders, R. J. and Warford, J. J. (1976). *Village water supply: economics and policy in the developing world.* Johns Hopkins University Press, Baltimore.

— Warford, J. J., and Mann, P. C. (1977). *Alternative concepts of marginal cost for public utility pricing: problems of application in the water supply sector.* Staff Working Paper No. 259. World Bank, Washington DC.

Scandizzo, P. L. and Knudsen, O. K. (1980). The evaluation of the benefits of basic need policies. *Am. J. agric. Econ.* **62**, 46–57.

Selowsky, M. (1979). *Who benefits from government expenditure? A case study of Colombia.* Oxford University Press, New York.

Shepard, D. S. and Zeckhauser, R. J. (1980). Long-term effects of interventions to improve survival in mixed populations. *J. chron. Dis.* **33**, 413–33.

Smith, J. (1980). *A review of the resources and service area of the health facilities in the Kingdom of Lesotho.* Ministry of Health, Maseru.

Squire, L. and Van der Tak, H. G. (1975). *Economic analysis of projects.* Johns Hopkins University Press, Baltimore.

Stolper, W. F. (1966). *Planning without facts.* Harvard University Press, Cambridge, Mass.

Streeten, P., Burki, S. J., Ul Haq, M., Hicks, N., and Stewart, F. (1981). *First things first: meeting basic human needs in developing countries.* Oxford University Press, New York.

Tait, A. A., Gratz, W. L. M., and Eichengreen, B. J. (1979). International comparisons of taxation for selected developing countries. *IMF Staff Pap.* **26**, 123–56.

Tan, E. A. (1975). Taxation, government spending and income distribution in the Philippines. Income Distribution and Employment Programme, Working Paper No. 26. International Labour Office, Geneva.

Thaler, R. and Rosen, S. (1975). The value of saving a life. In *Household production and consumption* (ed. N. E. Terleckyj). National Bureau of Economic Research, New York.

Torrance, G. W. (1976). Health status index models: a unified mathematical view. *Mgt Sci.* **22**, 990–1001.

Tuberculosis Prevention Trial (1979). Trial of BCG vaccines in South India for tuberculosis prevention: first report. *Bull. Wld Hlth Org.* **57**, 819–27.

Turvey, R. and Anderson, D. (1977). *Electricity economics: essays and case studies.* Johns Hopkins University Press, Baltimore.

Weisbrod, B. A. (1961). *Economics of public health: measuring the economic impact of diseases.* University of Pennsylvania Press, Philadelphia.

World Bank (1975). *Measurement of the health benefits of investments in water supply.* Public Utilities Report No. PUN 20. World Bank, Washington DC.

— (1981). *World development report 1981.* Oxford University Press, New York.

— (1982). *Malawi: growth and structural change, a basic economic report.* Report No. 3082–MAI. World Bank, Washington DC.

WHO (World Health Organization) (1977). *Financing of health services: report of a WHO study group. Tech. Rep. Ser. Wld Hlth Org.* **625**.

— (1981). Review of health expenditures, financial needs of the strategy for health for all by the year 2000, and the international flow of resources for the strategy. Document EB69/7. World Health Organization, Geneva.

Authors' note

The views and interpretations in this chapter are those of the authors and should not be attributed to the World Bank, to its affiliated organizations, or to any individual acting on their behalf.

8

The economic evaluation of immunization programmes

Andrew Creese

Introduction

Immunization as a primary health care activity has many advocates. The relative priority of any particular immunization programme in comparison with other life-saving investments in the health or allied sectors, and the question of how immunization may be delivered at least cost, are both, however, relatively unexplored areas. Both of these issues are central concerns of the health economist. This chapter illustrates, with reference to recent studies, how economic analysis is being employed in informing decisions about the desirability, scale, and organization of immunization programmes, and outlines what inadequacies exist and what improvements are needed in the analytical approaches used.

The section that follows gives some background to the epidemiology of communicable diseases in developing countries, and the special requirements for epidemiological data of health programme evaluation. The successful eradication of smallpox has no doubt been a major stimulus to increased support from international and bilateral agencies for immunization programmes. Besides being a preventive measure, immunization is directed at major sources of morbidity and mortality (particularly in infants); it has the capacity to be highly effective in reducing disease-specific morbidity and mortality rates; and it appears economical if one compares the cost per dose of vaccine with the price of routinely prescribed curative pharmaceuticals. Finally, since immunization involves a biochemical response, its success is not influenced by environmental and attitudinal factors beyond the decision to allow vaccination in the first place. Thus, unlike other low-cost primary health interventions such as health education directed at the safe disposal of solid waste, the ultimate success of immunization programmes does not depend on gradual social improvements. To this extent, immunization is a technical rather than a social approach to the problems of ill health in poor countries. Each of these apparent characteristics will be shown in what follows to be in need of further comment and qualification. To the present, however, the case for immunization has appeared sufficiently clear to obviate the need for extensive economic analysis, presumably on the (fallacious) grounds that any preventive measure is better than curative medicine (*Lancet* 1981). In fact, some of these very characteristics make it possible to pursue much further-reaching economic analysis of immunization programmes than is presently possible for other aspects of primary health care.

The availability of vaccines allows a well-defined set of alternative interventions to the standard curative responses to these diseases: immunization allows a choice of intervention time, rather like that allowed by the availability of diagnostic tests to screen for certain diseases, such as cervical cancer or Down's syndrome. Direct comparisons of the economic and epidemiological impact of immunization and non-immunization are therefore possible, and permit a comprehensive assessment of the issues involved in the decision whether to pursue a particular programme or not.

Several economic studies of immunization programmes have already been conducted in developed countries. As income levels increase in populations, the epidemiology of infectious diseases changes, age at first acquisition increasing and severity decreasing (though poliomyelitis is an exception to this pattern). The financial case for preventive programmes therefore changes as the costs of saving a life increase. A recent calculation of the costs and benefits of a schools BCG vaccination programme in Britain illustrated that (on the criterion of treatment savings alone) it is no longer economic, in view of the level of morbidity and treatment costs per case, to offer universal screening and vaccination to schoolchildren (Stilwell 1976). One of the major distinctions between the economics of immunization in developed and developing countries lies, therefore, in the epidemiology of the disease, which makes generalization from particular studies an unreliable basis for decision-making elsewhere. There are other differences, however, which necessitate special treatment in the economic evaluation of health programmes in LDCs, and these are discussed later (p. 151).

A number of choices face planners considering the establishment or enlargement of an immunization programme. The most general question is 'whether to undertake immunization?' and clearly the type of programme, its extent and location have to be specified before such a question may be answered. The underlying question here is 'is it worthwhile?' and the answer involves a cost–benefit approach to assess whether the resources deployed in a particular immunization programme generate enough gains in economic welfare to make the investment profitable. The notion of 'profitability' underpinning such studies is conceived much more widely than in commercial accounting terms or pure financial flows, and relates to the wider development objectives of the country in question (see Chapter 7). Such appraisal is seldom applied in health planning because of difficulties in measuring programme benefits, but it not only indicates the intrinsic value of a particular activity, but also allows it to be ranked in order of its investment priority with alternatives in the same or other sectors.

In specifying the nature of the programme, further choices have to be made. The geographical limits (if any), target age groups, vaccine type or combinations, vaccination schedules for multiple-dose immunization such as polio or DPT, all have to be specified and will all affect the final outcome of a cost–benefit appraisal. At present, few developing countries make all of the six common vaccinations universally available, so such choices are not hypothetical.

Issues of how a programme is to be specified influence whether it is likely to be socially and economically worthwhile; and further choices among alternative means can themselves be analysed by cost–effectiveness comparisons. Since the ultimate output of immunization is crudely measurable as lives saved, alternative programmes can be compared by estimating the costs per life saved by nutrition, water supply, or immunization interventions. Such studies are important in clarifying the range of alternative possible courses of action, which may include activities quite outside the health sector, and they escape some of the contentious issues in cost–benefit studies, most notably the valuation of measured performance. Cost–effectiveness comparisons are thus of use to decision-makers when the objective is both established and clearly specified. On p. 155 of this chapter, such analysis is referred to as inter-programme comparison.

Finally, even when a particular programme is selected as offering the least-cost method to the specified objective, there will remain intra-programme choices of optimal resource use. Questions as to the most efficient way to expand the programme in the light of existing coverage levels, possible combinations of fixed and mobile services of different types, and changing input prices will occur once the programme is operating, so that the *implementation* and management of a strategy will itself involve a series of choices, capable of yielding better or poorer performance from a given budget. On p. 162 these choices are discussed as intra-programme choices. The distinction between inter- and intra-programme choice is not intended to imply that such choices are necessarily *sequential*: different strategies of quite different programmes may be compared directly in cost-effectiveness terms (provided their effectiveness can be measured in identical units). Rather, the distinction is made to emphasize the availability of choices in a routine, managerial context, as well as in the pre-programme policy context.

Epidemiological factors

The most commonly available vaccines in the developing world are against tuberculosis (BCG), diphtheria, pertussis (whooping cough), and tetanus, and to a lesser extent, against measles and poliomyelitis. Vaccines also exist, or are in the developmental stage, against many other diseases such as yellow fever, rubella (German measles), influenza, cholera, typhoid, mumps, meningitis, leprosy, and malaria. Accurate estimates of the incidence in developing countries of tuberculosis, measles, poliomyelitis, diphtheria, pertussis, and tetanus are hard to obtain and the reported rates (see Table 8.1) are certainly under-estimates, for survey-based estimates show how much higher actual rates are than reported cases, and how heavily concentrated the cases are in the very young. Globally, the World Health Organization assesses the incidence of measles at close to 100 per cent of children surviving to the age of 9 months, with case fatality rates of between 2 per cent and 8 per cent. Some 80 per cent of children are estimated to get pertussis before reaching 5 years, with case fatality rates of between 1 per cent and 3 per cent. Surveys in Bangladesh, India, and Indonesia

TABLE 8.1 *Reported incidence rates per 100 000 population 1974–1978 (world)*

	1974	1978
Measles	95	95
TB	85	70
Pertussis	35	50
Tetanus	5.8	4.0
Diphtheria	1.8	2.2
Polio	1.2	1.3

Adapted from *Weekly Epidemiological Record* 21, 156, Fig. 3 (1980).

indicate a neonatal tetanus incidence rate of about 15 per 1000 live births, with a case fatality rate in excess of 85 per cent.

A recent study in Kenya used the estimates of age-specific incidence shown in Table 8.2. With estimated case-fatality rates at age 1 of 0.2 for diptheria, tetanus, and tuberculosis, 1.183 for polio, and 0.118 for measles, the mortality impact of these diseases can be seen as substantial. On these estimates, substantially over 3000 of every 100000 one-year olds would die from one of these diseases in any year. On a world-wide basis, WHO estimate that some five million children die from these diseases each year.

TABLE 8.2. *Estimated incidence rates per 100 000 by age—Kenya, 1979*

Age	0–1 yr	1–2 yrs	2–3 yrs
Measles	14700	25500	15600
TB	150	150	150
Pertussis	15800	9700	13900
Tetanus	12000	300	300
Diphtheria	50	200	100
Polio	61	66	65

Source: Barnum 1980.

Programme effectiveness may be judged by the extent of the reduction in the number of cases of a particular disease occurring in a defined population; but since good data on both incidence rates and population denominators for developing countries are frequently lacking, the number of *vaccinated individuals* is often used as a basis for estimating numbers of cases prevented (WHO 1977). Such estimates necessitate the use of an overall index of vaccine efficacy, and these values in turn are commonly based on historical averages, such as the pre- and post-pertussis immunization incidence rates for England and Wales (DHSS 1977). Recent WHO estimates of efficacy for infant immunizations are shown in Table 8.3.

Several important potential 'leakages' from these high overall levels of efficacy may lower the actual impact of immunization programmes, however. The *quality of vaccine as manufactured* differs from country to country, and sometimes from batch to batch. National vaccine quality control facilities are

TABLE 8.3. *Vaccine efficacy for infants*

Measles	95%	
Pertussis	80%	(as component of three-dose DPT immunizations, given at least four weeks apart)
Poliomyelitis	95%	(efficacy of three doses trivalent OPV, at least four weeks apart)
Diphtheria	99%	
Tuberculosis	80%	

Adapted from WHO, *Indicators and targets for the expanded programme on immunization*, EPI/GEN/81/2.

still the exception rather than the rule: in 1980 there was only one DPT quality control facility in all Africa and only two measles vaccine control facilities in Central and South America. Furthermore, of the 25 per cent of countries for which complete information on vaccine quality existed for DPT, BCG, measles and poliomyelitis, one fifth were using vaccines which did not comply with World Health Organization requirements on quality. Further, even vaccine of known quality may fail to produce the intended immunological response. Well conducted trials of BCG immunization have shown efficacy to range from zero to 80 per cent and the reasons for such divergence remain unclear. Glassroth, Robins, and Snider (1980) recognize 'potency and immunogenecity of the vaccine, sensitisation of the vaccinated population by non-tuberculous mycobacteria, the nutritional status of the vaccinated population and many other factors' as contributory. Differences in sero-conversion rates, which provide a measure of the immunity in the vaccinated individual, mean that total numbers vaccinated may misrepresent the actual number of cases prevented, so serological surveys are necessary to establish whether a satisfactory antibody response has been achieved. Such information not only assists with the measurement of programme performance, but also allows the identification of the most responsive section of the population, as Henderson (1981) has shown in identifying the optimal age of measles vaccination in Kenya as eight to ten months.

A major managerial problem relevant to effective vaccination is the maintenance of vaccine potency by freezing or refrigeration of vaccines and ensuring that their shelf life is not excessive. Whilst the stability of vaccines under different temperature regimes is still under investigation, it is clear that for all vaccines potency is reduced by prolonged storage at high temperatures. The operation of a continuous *cold chain* to keep vaccines at appropriate temperatures (4–8 °C for DPT/BCG; −20–+8 °C for OPV and measles vaccine) is therefore of great importance, and problematic where extensive transportation in hot conditions is necessary. Related managerial failures which could reduce programme effectiveness involve misidentifying non-immunized 'target' age group children; inappropriate sterilization and quantities of vaccine; and failure to explain the importance of follow-up vaccinations. The Expanded Programme on Immunization of WHO, with support from UNDP and UNICEF, is tackling these problems in a variety of ways and improving both the design of material for developing country conditions and the managerial capacity of primary health workers.

Improving immunization programme effectiveness, therefore, involves a knowledge of the way vaccination raises the level of immunity of the individuals (and the population); and this requires serological survey, careful quality control at the vaccine production stage, and the maintenance of an effective cold chain from factory to health unit. Little quantitative evidence exists on the importance of these individual sources of reduction in total programme effectiveness and there are obvious limitations on the use of developed country experience in those matters.

Economic analysis of cost per life saved or case prevented by immunization, as discussed in the following sections, is therefore inevitably built on cruder assumptions than are ideal; but this is in large measure because the epidemiological data are frequently suspect, absent, or contradictory.

Cost–benefit analysis (CBA) of immunization programmes

The total number of cost–benefit studies of immunization, whether in developed or developing countries, is small; and there is a considerable diversity in the approaches taken. Basically, these differences reduce to different degrees of comprehensiveness and of accuracy in the measurement of programme costs and benefits, and reflect the demanding requirements of a full cost–benefit approach to programme evaluation. The essential requirement of CBA in immunization is that the present value of real resource use occasioned by the programme be compared with the value of the programme's output. Real resource use involves the value of the labour and capital equipment needed to deliver vaccinations and the costs borne by the vaccinee and family (such as travel costs and work time foregone in travelling and waiting). Such costs may need to be valued on a different basis from the market prices for individual components, as Chapter 7 illustrates, and costs may need to be attributed (as with patients' foregone work or leisure) where no prices exist.

The benefits of immunization are easier to identify than to measure or value. They consist essentially of the avoided costs of disease, which are usually understood to include:

direct costs—public and private expenditures occasioned in the treatment of disease and rehabilitation; and
indirect costs of two kinds—those involving losses in production and productive capacity, typically the economic consequences of morbidity and premature mortality from disease; and those involving losses in 'utility' or general well-being, such as anxiety, pain, discomfort, and bereavement.

In the case of communicable diseases, there is another important item of benefit: external economies in consumption. Third party welfare losses are reduced by each individual decision to vaccinate children by reduction of the general risk of contagion; so that the benefits to the community at risk are greater than the sum of the individual benefits from vaccination. There is thus some element of disease costs avoided for persons other than the individual choosing vaccination, for the same categories as above, and this should, in principle, be enumerated and valued as a component of benefit. Analogously, an optimal level of vaccination in a particular community may well be at less than 100 per cent of the population vulnerable to the disease. Finally, where the government has clear redistributional objectives, such as implied in the 'basic needs' approach, these can be reflected in the economic analysis by a system of differential weights, so that no conflict exists between explicit intentions of the government and actual plans.

Review of some cost-benefit studies

Most studies of immunization in developing countries neglect some of these requirements. For instance, the cost–benefit 'balance point' proposed in the methodology of Grab and Cvjetanovic (1977) is concerned with the relationship between only vaccination costs and treatment cost savings, neglecting the indirect, but ultimately more important, gains in health status of the population. Barnum, Tarantola, and Setiady (1980) make similar comparisons of immunization costs and potential treatment savings in what is principally a cost–effectiveness analysis of DPT/BCG vaccination in Indonesia.

No account is taken in the methodology of Grab and Cvejtanovic of private expenditures on treatment, though Barnum's study estimates these. Such payments are substantial in many countries, and they contain direct evidence of individuals' valuations of the reduction in risk resulting from immunization. Since the 'treatment savings in the public sector' approach omits individual and social valuations of reduced morbidity and mortality, it cannot in isolation be used as a basis for decision-making about the net social value of immunizations *unless this appears to be positive.* If the savings in public sector treatment outlays are big enough to offset the costs of the immunization programme, as Burgasov *et al.* (1973) argued in the case of the mass immunization against measles programme in the USSR, then the programme is economically worthwhile. Unfortunately, one of the principal objectives of CBA is frustrated by this approach: by not knowing *how* worthwhile (i.e. by how much the benefits from the programme outweigh its costs), it is not possible to rank order immunization against other life-saving investments. Whilst an excess of the value of benefits over costs is a *necessary* condition for any investment, it is not a *sufficient* condition.

In an earlier paper, Barnum (AID 1978) undertook a comparison in Indonesia of the costs of BCG and/or DPT vaccination with benefits assessed in terms of treatment savings, productivity gains and savings in mothers' time spent in home care. This study was one of the first to consider the opportunity cost of foreign exchange and unskilled labour inputs in an immunization appraisal. For example, it derived a shadow price or value for female labour based on female participation rates, market wages and seasonal employment opportunities. This value (31 per cent of the average wage rate for unskilled labour) was then used to estimate the value of maternal time spent per case in caring for sick infants—the saving of which constitutes one of the categories of benefit from immunization. Discounted future earnings, with an allowance for productivity growth, were the basis for Barnum's estimates of productivity benefits from reduced mortality; though no value was attached to morbidity reductions or the pure utility gains associated with infant disease reduction. External benefits were not itemized, but a sensitivity analysis was undertaken. Barnum's study indicated that, considered as a separate programme, BCG immunization showed a benefit:cost ratio of 1.48:1 but that this positive net present value was not robust to plausible changes in the principal cost and benefit parameters. DPT immunization as a separate programme showed a higher benefit:cost ratio of 2.4:1 and the combined programmes a ratio of 2.9:1, and Barnum concluded:

Even when the costs are increased by 20% and the benefits decreased by 33%, the ratio of benefits to costs remains greater than one and the net present value positive. Clearly, the total project is economically viable and desirable.

Methodologically, Barnum's study is an important advance over the Grab and Cvejtanovic work and it is, at present, the most comprehensive analysis of the 'economic' case for BCG and DPT vaccination in a developing country.

In a cost–benefit analysis of measles immunization in Southern Zambia, Pönnighaus (1979) documents how the programme changes its economic character as more dispersed rural populations are included. For the most favourable urban setting, the present value of benefits exceeded the costs by 4.4:1 but this benefit–cost ratio fell to 4.4:16 for full coverage of the most dispersed rural population. The Pönnighaus study does not consider user cost savings or external benefits, and it places no value on the utility gain from the increased probability of survival, but it does impute a productivity loss of about K150 (£112) per premature death. This study documents how rapidly the costs of vaccinating additional infants may rise, but the policy conclusions drawn about the overall 'economic' case for measles immunization (i.e. that it is worthwhile in urban areas with 24-hour electricity but not in rural areas with scattered populations) seem, on the basis of the data presented, open to question. The total costs of immunization and approximate number of lives saved, according to Pönnighaus's data, are shown in Table 8.4.

Programme benefits are estimated as follows in Table 8.5. Using minimum estimates of life-saving thus gives the following benefits for each location (Table 8.6). So, on these minimum estimates, a positive benefit–cost ratio of 1.27:1 emerges. Using the maximum rates of life-saving in each location raises this ratio to 2.33:1, giving an overall benefit:cost ratio of 1.8:1.

If the investment question is of the form 'is it worth immunizing children against measles?' then the Pönnighaus study shows that, overall, it is; with a benefit–cost ratio of approximately 1.8:1. However, Pönnighaus is not concerned

TABLE 8.4. *Measles immunization in southern Zambia*

Location	Total cost (Kwacha)	Approx. no. lives saved
Monze town	444	13–23
Namwala township	237	3–6
Namwala district (75% cover)	2754.8	15–27
Namwala district (remaining 25% cover)	2934.8	5–10
Total	3670.6	36–66

Source: Pönnighaus 1979.

TABLE 8.5. *Benefits in relation to one life probably saved in Monze and Namwala towns and in Namwala district for 75 per cent and 100 per cent coverage offered*

	Monze town	Namwala town	Namwala district (75%)	Namwala district (other 25%)
Saved treatment costs	↑	K32.95 to K132	↓	↓↓
Avoided loss to economy	K150	K150	K150	K150
Benefits	↑	K183 to K282	↓	↓↓

Economic benefits compared to Namwala town
↑ more ↓ less ↓↓ much less

Source: Pönnighaus 1979.

TABLE 8.6. *Total benefits of measles immunization by district*

Monze town	13 lives × (150 + 82.5)	= 3022.5 (underestimate of benefit)
Namwala town	3 lives × (150 + 82.5)	= 697.5
Namwala district (75%)	15 lives × (150 + 82.5)	= 3487.5 (overestimate of benefit)
Namwala district (other 25%)	5 lives × (150 + 32.95)	= 914.75
		8122.25 total benefit

to make this point, but to document the *different* cost-benefit ratios for different sections of the population. It could be argued that this is to place too heavy reliance on cost-benefit analysis. What the Pönnighaus study shows is that measles vaccination *is* worthwhile (on his own assumptions) even when, for a substantial proportion of the population, the benefit–cost ratio is unfavourable. The study demonstrates how a methodology that assigns equal weight to all individuals will lead to an unequal distribution of resources in favour of urban areas. The analysis is sound, but unnecessarily limited: instead, differential weights could have been attached to different socioeconomic or geographical sections of the total population to re-examine the viability of the entire project.

A study by Makinen (1979) in Yaoundé, Cameroon provides what is probably the most comprehensive cost-benefit study of measles immunization to date. This takes account of private as well as public expenditures in both vaccinating infants (costs), and in reduced time spent caring for sick children (benefit). Corrections are made to local market prices for foreign exchange and unskilled labour inputs, though it is unclear whether these modifications affect the conclusions substantially. The value of external benefits to measles vaccination is incorporated, using a modified version of the Reed-Frost model of measles case transmission. Makinen's conclusions are tested for their sensitivity to a variety of assumptions about the value of parental time, the case fatality rate, discount rate, and growth rate in productivity, but no direct estimate of the utility gains from immunization is attempted. On most conservative assumptions the programme is economically strongly worthwhile, with an overall benefit-cost ratio of at least 25.3:1, indicating an unusually high rate of return from this investment. Makinen comments:

Measles vaccinations in Yaoundé appear to be an overwhelmingly favourable project, no matter what restrictions are placed on benefits. This result suggests that there may be a broad under-allocation of funds to health projects, so that wider application of benefit–cost analysis to health programmes may result in bigger health budgets, hence better health.

Comparing the above studies in terms of their economic methodology, it is apparent that considerable divergence of practice exists; and also that empirical work shows positive—often high—net present values for all programmes. The only evidence of an overall immunization programme being not economically worthwhile is Stilwell's study of school BCG vaccination in Britain (Stilwell 1976). In general, contemporary studies suggest that attack rates, vaccination effectiveness, and gains in productivity are sufficiently high, and costs sufficiently low for immunization programmes to be worthwhile over a wide range of developing country conditions, particularly for measles, DPT, and BCG, though the insecure epidemiological foundations which underpin working assumptions about effectiveness (p. 148) should be remembered.

Cost-effectiveness comparisons of immunization and alternative primary health care strategies

Cost-effectiveness analyses (CEAs) may be employed in decision-making in a range of different ways. Such analyses take the desirability of the programme objectives as given (unlike in CBA, which attempts to assess precisely this); and are concerned to identify the most economically efficient way to achieve these objectives. This section reviews existing evidence on the cost-effectiveness of alternative methods of reducing infant mortality. These studies are not necessarily disease specific: they are concerned with *inter*-programme choice;

and consider such different interventions as water supply improvement, oral rehydration, or nutrition programmes, as well as different immunization programmes. The comparisons are thus among programmes whose final effect may be measured in common (mortality) terms, but which may involve preventive or curative interventions of either a disease-specific or a multipurpose nature. The operational importance of such studies is, of course, substantial from a planning viewpoint, as they aim to identify the least-cost route to saving a specified number of lives. In most studies, the decision criterion is a simple ratio of cost to effectiveness; and in the appraisal of mutually exclusive projects, this is clearly adequate. From the viewpoint of *programme balance*, however, where national health planners may require information about which programmes to emphasize or scale down, and where within a wide range programmes will be complementary to each other, the information required on cost–effectiveness should relate to *marginal* changes in performance, i.e. the ratio of an increase in costs to an increase in effectiveness for each programme.

Several measures of effectiveness have been employed in the studies reviewed, ranging from costs per vaccination or costs per fully vaccinated infant, through to estimates of cost per case or death prevented. The last is the closest approximation to a measure of final health output for a programme. Table 8.7 illustrates its calculation.

TABLE 8.7. *Number of lives saved by immunization*

$$L_i = \sum_i N_i A_i (do_i - d_i)$$

where L_i = lives saved in age group i
N_i = numbers of fully immunized in age group i
A_i = disease and age-specific attack rate
do_i = disease and age-specific mortality rate without immunization
d_i = disease and age-specific mortality rate with immunization

The earliest such study was a comparison of the relative cost–effectiveness of immunization and hospitalization in Morocco (Barlow 1976). This estimated the cost per life saved in different types of hospital and by different vaccination programmes and established firstly that vaccination is a more cost–effective method of saving lives than hospital care, and secondly that DPT/BCG programmes are more economically efficient than immunization against poliomyelitis. However, the study did not actually compare comparable cases in the two interventions, as it looked at the costs of preventing a death *for all patients* in hospital; so it documents in the most general way the potential economies of primary preventive intervention against secondary or tertiary curative care. No account was taken in this study of the adequacy of using agency costs alone (neglecting, in particular, user and user-family costs); nor of the possibility of price corrections being necessary for any of the inputs to the hospital or vaccination programme. The external benefits to vaccination programmes were not taken into account in the comparison.

TABLE 8.8. *Cost-effectiveness of possible immunization programmes for Kenya, 1979*

Programme	Cost/death prevented (US $)
DPT, TT, BCG only	274
DPT, TT, BCG as marginal programme	69
Measles only	50
Measles as marginal programme	26
Polio only	6357
Polio as marginal programme	568
Total programme	85

Source: Barnum 1980.

Contemporary concerns have concentrated more narrowly on establishing priorities among *primary* interventions, and in a study based on Kenya, Barnum (1980) has compared the costs per death prevented with different immunization programmes, with oral rehydration treatment for diarrhoeal disease, and with a low technology water supply project. Barnum distinguishes between the costs of preventing a death by immunization according to whether the immunization in question is the basic or marginal component of the programme (the incremental costs of introducing new vaccines being less than the launching costs of a programme). The results appear in Table 8.8. From Table 8.8, it can be seen that poliomyelitis life-saving is relatively costly, a consequence of the lower incidence and case fatality rate of this disease, whereas measles vaccination appears to be the most cost–effective way of saving life if a single immunization programme were to be chosen. However, the total programme cost-per-life-saved shows that additional immunization may be given at little additional cost, suggesting that, in practice, a multiple antigen immunization programme would be preferred.

The study acknowledges that cost–effectiveness comparisons of immunization with either oral rehydration or community water supply projects is hampered because the effectiveness of immunizations is more firmly established than for the other projects. None the less, estimates are provided of costs per death prevented at different levels of programme effectiveness, effectiveness in all cases being measured in terms of the reduction in case fatality rate. The data suggests that polio immunization alone is likely to be the least cost–effective intervention with a cost per death prevented of $568. Public water provision, even at maximum effectiveness, has an estimated cost per death prevented of $230 and is therefore less cost–effective than the total immunization programme where the estimated cost per death prevented is $85. If oral rehydration is fully effective (saving the maximum possible number of lives), costs per death prevented by this method are approximately $30, making this *potentially* the most cost–effective intervention. However, the likely effectiveness of oral rehydration therapy is subject to considerable variation and at a 40 per cent effectiveness level the cost per prevented death is identical with that of the total immunization programme. Barnum's is an important study in comparing choices in primary health care, by examining the way cost–effectiveness changes with different assumptions about the effectiveness of projects. In addition, quite apart from its methodological improvement over the earlier Barlow study, it compares interventions with health consequences that may be the responsibility of quite different agencies, thus recognizing that health planning choices in developing countries may well be wider than the options which the health sector itself can offer. Overall, though, the relative cost–effectiveness of immunizations, and the degree of firmness in these estimates, still makes such programmes likely priorities. A similar study by Grosse (1980) made tentative estimates of the consequences of alternative health promotion strategies in regions of Indonesia, Pakistan, and Ghana; and suggested that the mortality and morbidity improvements from additional immunization and nutrition programmes may be greater than for sanitation programmes.

TABLE 8.9. *Cost-effectiveness of the proposed immunization programme*

	Cost per death prevented (Rp)	Cost per case prevented (Rp)	Cost of treating one case* (Rp)
Total programme	53963	3942	13166
BCG programme only	188623 (US $455)	42438	49000
DPTT programme only	55905 (US $135)	3679	11459
BCG considered as an added programme	42043 (US $101)	9459	49000
DPTT considered as an added programme	32027 (US $77)	2107	11459
Total programme in last year of plan (1983–4)	50750 (US $122)	3620	13166

*This is the weighted average of the costs of treatment of the diseases considered. The weights are the proportions of total prevented cases in each disease category.
Source: Barnum *et al.* 1980.

A recent study by Barnum and colleagues (1980) compares the cost–effectiveness of alternative immunization strategies in Indonesia, the results of which are summarized in Table 8.9. DPTT vaccination as a separate programme is seen as more cost-effective than BCG, in contrast with Barlow's findings for Morocco. Since differences in programme effectiveness within the two countries are greater than internal cost differences between the programmes, and since similar vaccine effectiveness rates are used in both studies, the explanation for this difference in cost–effectiveness must lie in Morocco's substantially higher tuberculosis death rate. Unfortunately, how much of this is attributable to greater incidence and how much to greater case-fatality is impossible to determine from the data of the Moroccan study.

A related logic to that of cost–benefit/cost–effectiveness appraisal is contained in the *priority-scaling* approach, first proposed in the context of personal social services programmes by Algie and Miller (1976) and subsequently evident in the *Country Health Programming* approach of WHO. To take account of the 'epidemiological' character of the problems facing social services agencies, as well as the effectiveness and cost of available services, Algie and Miller proposed combining quantitative information about:

— the nature and scale of each of the principal problems facing the agency;
— the available service responses for these problems
— the estimated impacts of these responses, and
— agency resource costs.

No particular method was suggested for combining these ingredients in making decisions, but the similarity of procedure to a cost–effectiveness approach is apparent.

Variants of this approach have subsequently been used in setting health sector priorities in the developing world. Walsh and Warren (1979), using four priority criteria of prevalence, mortality, morbidity, and feasibility of control, and assigning ordinal values (e.g. high, extremely low) to each of 24 disease groups, assigned each disease to an overall priority group. The actual details of the measurement and aggregation procedure used in this study are unclear— relative weights for each of the four criteria are not disclosed and the precise scales used in measuring each of the diseases in terms of these criteria are not discussed. Further, the procedure contains a substantial amount of implicit reasoning, for example, in assessing 'feasibility of control'. The authors claim that such an approach constitutes 'the beginnings of a cost-effectiveness analysis', however; and in their attempt to be *comprehensive* and consistent in comparing estimated production relationships on a disease-by-disease basis, this is probably correct. Immunization against measles, whooping cough, and neonatal tetanus emerge in the 'high' priority group and, since the marginal cost of diphtheria and BCG vaccination has been shown to be small in other studies, this would presumably establish immunization against the commonest childhood diseases (with the exception of poliomyelitis), as a high priority. It should be noted that, for operational purposes, the ordinal priority index allows no interpretation of the degree to which malnutrition, for instance, is more important than Chagas' disease; or whether the same degree of difference in priorities obtains between all diseases. However, the purpose of the study was illustrative rather than operational.

Use of the same basic approach was made in preparing the 1979–83 health plan in the People's Democratic Republic of Yemen (1979). The criteria for disease priority are shown in Table 8.10 and each criterion was assigned a relative weight. Each disease was then scored on a five-point scale and an aggregate weighted score calculated to give a cardinal index of priority (see

TABLE 8.10. *Weighted criteria used in priority scaling of health programmes, People's Democratic Republic of Yemen*

Criteria	Relative weight
A. Availability of technology	3
B. Morbidity	2
C. Mortality	2
D. Effect on economy (productivity)	2
E. Cost of disease	2
F. Political and public concern	2
G. Disease predisposition—sequelae contribution to other diseases	2
H. Contagiousness and potential for epidemic outbreak	2

Scoring scale
4:    extremely high
3:    high
2:    medium
1:    low
0:    negligible

Source: People's Democratic Republic of Yemen, Five-Year Health Plan, 1979-83 (1979).

Table 8.11). As can be seen, communicable childhood diseases (immunization programme) emerged as the clear top priority.

Though these latter exercises are not strictly cost-effectiveness studies, their general approach and purpose is to identify the 'best' pattern of expenditure. This is defined with reference to the epidemiology of the diseases, the technical effectiveness of control or preventive measures and their cost. In addition, to make the ranking process work, valuations by decision-makers are introduced to specify the relative importance of the principal criteria and the actual values attached to each disease. The general method, aiming at a consistent and explicit basis for the comparison of alternative claims on the limited resources of the health sector, is therefore essentially that of cost–effectiveness, applied at the highest level of priority setting. Earlier reference to such methodological considerations as non-agency costs (e.g. to users of the service and to non-Ministry of Health providers); efficiency price corrections in the light of foreign exchange values and domestic unemployment rates; and equity corrections in the light of the income and regional location of populations should all be included in such studies as also should considerations of the *marginal* impact of expansion/contraction in individual programmes.

In this section a number of studies have been identified that compare the cost-effectiveness of different immunization programmes and of alternative interventions to reduce infant mortality. The existing evidence on programme effectiveness is rather stronger for immunizations than for other programmes, though there is considerable variation in the estimated costs of preventing a death by a given programme, reflecting differences in the incidence and case-fatality rates,

TABLE 8.11. *People's Democratic Republic of Yemen: health sector priorities*

Disease	Priority	Total score	A		B		C		D		E		F		G		H	
			S	S×W	S	S×W	S	S×W	S	S×W	S	S×W	S	S×W	S	S×W	S	S×W
Common childhood infections (immunization)	(1)	53	3	9	3	6	3	6	2	4	3	6	4	8	3	6	4	8
Malaria	(2)	48	4	12	3	6	2	4	3	6	2	4	3	6	3	6	2	4
Diarrhoeal diseases	(3)	47	3	9	3	6	3	6	2	4	3	6	3	6	3	6	2	4
Other respiratory infections (excluding TB)	(4)	42	2	6	3	6	3	6	3	6	2	4	1	2	3	6	3	6
TB	(5)	41	3	9	3	6	2	4	3	6	3	6	3	6	1	2	1	2
Anaemia	(6)	40	3	9	2	4	1	2	2	4	3	6	2	4	3	6	1	2
Malnutrition (PEM)	(7)	38	2	6	2	4	2	4	2	4	3	6	3	6	3	6	1	2
Schistosomiasis	(8)	36	2	4	3	6	2	4	3	6	1	2	3	6	2	4	1	2
Infectious eye diseases including trachoma	(9)	35	3	9	3	6	0	–	2	4	3	6	2	4	1	2	2	4
Perinatal morbidity and mortality	(9)	35	3	9	2	4	2	4	1	2	2	4	3	6	2	4	1	2

Key: S = Score; W = Relative weight.
Source: People's Democratic Republic of Yemen, Five-Year Plan, 1979–83 (1979).

and also variations in vaccine effectiveness in the field. Overall, priority-scaling exercises and empirical work indicate that immunization with measles, DPT and BCG have very high relative priority *vis-à-vis* other health programmes; and Barnum's study in Kenya indicates that immunization is overall likely to be more cost-effective than a water-supply project. However, poliomyelitis immunization appears to be a less cost-effective intervention than others, and recent evaluations of the effect of BCG and measles vaccination on immune status in India and Zaïre suggest that there may be some over-estimation of the potential of these antigens. There is a possibility that oral rehydration interventions may be still more cost-effective than immunization, though there is currently little firm evidence on this.

Cost-effectiveness analysis within immunization programmes

The challenge to maximize value for money continues to apply within established immunization programmes as well as to the initial investment choices between programmes. Wherever alternative ways of providing immunizations exist, the basic notions of cost-effectiveness comparing incremental costs with incremental effect, measured in lives saved or simply as children immunized, may be employed. Such alternatives are numerous. Many programmes pursue several different strategies simultaneously and thereby offer operational evidence of the relative cost–effectiveness of each. Different vaccines, different vaccination schedules, different combinations of fixed centre or mobile outreach facilities, different degrees of integration with existing basic health services, and different types of immunization personnel are all examples of the alternative choices open to immunization programme managers. Questions of cost-effective programme performance arise during the operation of the programme, therefore, and there is a need for managers of immunization programmes (in common with health planners) to be acquainted with the basic notions of economic decision-making (EPI 1980*a*).

Barnum's cost–effectiveness study in Kenya addressed the problem faced *within* the immunization programme of whether or not to immunize the 'backlog' of non-immunized children aged up to five, inherited before the programme began (Barnum 1980). A choice faces programme managers in all countries on the launching or augmentation of immunization services whether, given limited budgets, to vaccinate only newborn infants or children at risk ages in the population as well. Barnum compared the costs per life saved from offering vaccination to newborns and older children, and showed that the higher attack rates and case-fatality rates in the first year or so of life made it possible to maximize the number of lives saved by concentrating the programme on newborn infants. He concluded:

While the absolute difference in cost is not great . . . the cost differential does imply that, if financial restraints limited the adoption of the entire programme it would be more cost-effective to concentrate on immunisation of newborns for a larger area rather than the addition of an immunisation programme for older children to an existing newborn programme for a smaller area.

Such formal analysis may be simple, even rough; but it is clearly necessary to assist decision-making.

For many developing countries, it will remain important that comparisons between different immunization strategies should make use of the shadow pricing procedures outlined earlier. This point can be illustrated by reference to the World Health Organization/Government of Ghana Pilot Studies of an Expanded Programme of Immunization, 1976-78 (Litvinov *et al.* 1979). Immunization was offered by both fully mobile and limited outreach teams in two regions of Ghana; and the financial costs of the immunizing units were as given in Table 8.12. However, both strategies involved the use of some imported inputs and thus foreign exchange at a time when the official exchange rate of the Ghana *cedi* heavily overrated its value (Barnett, Creese, and Ayivor 1980). Table 8.13 shows recalculated total costs when the foreign exchange components of both types of health centre are shadow priced so as to represent the 'true' cost of foreign exchange, conservatively approximated at 2.5 times the official rate.

TABLE 8.12. *Financial cost per fully immunized infant, 1976-1978*

		Cedis
Region 1	Mobile Field Team 1	10.8
	Fixed Centre Team A	40.7
	Fixed Centre Team B	37.04
	Fixed Centre Team C	35.10
	Fixed Centre Team D	36.96
Region 2	Mobile Field Team 2	12.83
	Fixed Centre Team E	12.92
	Fixed Centre Team F	90.23
	Fixed Centre Team G	33.94
	Fixed Centre Team H	40.36

Source: Litvinov *et al.* 1979.

Not only do the 'true' costs of immunization appear substantially higher when overvaluation of the domestic currency is taken into account, but the rank order of cost–effectiveness changes; for instance, in Region 2, the mobile unit is no longer the most cost-effective.

Such price corrections are important when programmes with differing proportions of imported inputs, or differing combination of skilled and unskilled labour, are being considered. The general effect of shadow pricing will be to emphasize the relative merits of those options using the greatest proportions of low-skilled labour and domestically produced material inputs. In conjunction with redistributive guidelines, government concern to promote the welfare of low-income groups can also be incorporated into such cost-effectiveness

TABLE 8.13. *Economic cost per fully immunized infant, 1976-1978*

		Cedis
Region 1	Mobile Field Team 1	17.43
	Fixed Centre Team A	56.16
	Fixed Centre Team B	52.60
	Fixed Centre Team C	46.74
	Fixed Centre Team D	56.65
Region 2	Mobile Field Team 2	20.09
	Fixed Centre Team E	19.51
	Fixed Centre Team F	144.38
	Fixed Centre Team G	54.81
	Fixed Centre Team H	65.48

comparisons, thus reducing the apparent undesirability of rural immunization activity indicated in the study by Pönnighaus above (p. 153). More widely, the development of guidelines on shadow prices, and promotion of a common set of practices for valuing project inputs and outputs, would enable health sector decisions to be made on a basis consistent with the development objectives of other sectors, such as agriculture, water supply, and transportation.

Decisions on the geographical areas to be covered by the programme, on the expansion to new areas or increased coverage within existing areas, can be assessed rapidly in cost–effectiveness terms on the assumption that the objective is the maximization of the number of fully immunized infants. From data on the rate at which costs increase with, for example, population density or other measures of 'accessibility', it may then be possible to identify *thresholds* or switching points in the programme at which the least-cost delivery method changes from, say, static units to mobile ones.

In the development of national and international management skills for immunization programmes, the World Health Organization's Expanded Programme on Immunization (EPI) promotes the use of simplified cost-effectiveness measures in routine programme audit. Guidelines for estimating costs per fully immunized infant have been produced and field tested in a small number of countries, and provide descriptive information on the distribution of programme costs between capital and operating costs, and on sub-categories of operating cost such as vaccines, health centre staff costs, supervision and training costs, cold chain costs, transportation, etc., at small samples of health centres (EPI 1980*a*). Such estimates provide an initial basis for comparisons between rural and urban programmes and large or small health units; and for considering or rejecting modifications to the programme in the form of staffing, deployment of supervisory resources, or use of vehicles. Preliminary studies have identified overstaffing in relation to actual workloads of vaccinators in Indonesia (EPI 1981), and inefficiency resulting from low utilization rates at some rural health centres in Thailand (EPI 1980*b*).

Conclusions

The economic evaluation of immunization programmes involves first identifying choices at several levels of decision-making and then conducting an analysis of resource use and programme yield associated with each choice. The most general questions are of the cost–benefit form and ask whether the programme should be undertaken at all. The results of some attempts to answer this question in developing countries have been discussed. Cost–benefit studies of immunization, such as those by Makinen and Pönnighaus, suggest that not only is measles vaccination worthwhile as a health activity, but also that it compares favourably with the rates of return obtainable in other sectors of the economy, including those more usually thought of as conventionally 'productive'. Additional vaccines may therefore be economically worthwhile because of their low marginal cost.

The next level in decision-making is that of comparison among a number of alternative means to an accepted end, that of saving lives. In this type of comparison, the objective itself is not at issue; the problem is to identify the least-cost strategy. This may either involve comparisons of immunization with selected other programmes, or it may be a part of a much wider attempt to establish local or national disease priorities on an inter-programme basis. Again, existing evidence indicates a high priority for infant immunization as among the most cost-effective health interventions, though substantially more empirical work is required in this area.

At the lowest level is decision-making of a managerial, continuous kind. The concern here is to identify and maintain the maximum performance from the programme budget. Economic work in this area is still in its infancy and its growth will ultimately depend on the wider use of simple economic principles in the management of the health sector as a whole. All three types of appraisal are complementary and essential; the techniques are in principle relatively simple; and the result of their application is increased consistency and explicitness in project and programme decision-making.

REFERENCES

AID (Agency for International Development) (1978). *Indonesia—expanded programme on immunisation* AID/BAS–014, Washington DC.
Algie, J. and Miller, C. (1976). Deciding social service priorities. *J. appl. Systems Analysis* 5, 29–48.
Barlow, R. (1976). Applications of a health planning model in Morocco. *Int. J. Hlth Serv.* 6, 103–22.
Barnett, A., Creese, A. L., and Ayivor, E. C. K. (1980). The economics of pharmaceuticals policy in Ghana. *Int. J. Hlth Serv.* 10, 479–99.
Barnum, H. N. (1980). Cost-effectiveness of programs to combat communicable childhood diseases in Kenya. (Mimeo.) Agency for International Development, Washington, DC.
— Tarantola, I. F., and Setiady, I. F. (1980). Cost-effectiveness of an immunisation programme in Indonesia. *Bull. Wld Hlth Org.* 58, 499–503.
Burgasov, P. N., Andzaparidze, O. G., and Popov, V. F. (1973). The status of measles after 5 years of mass vaccination in the U.S.S.R. *Bull. Wld Hlth Org.* 49, 571.

DHSS (Department of Health and Social Security) (1977). *Whooping cough vaccination: Review of the evidence on whooping cough vaccination by the joint committee on vaccination and immunisation.* HMSO, London.

EPI (Expanded Programme Immunization) (1980a). Programme costing guidelines. *Weekly Epidemiol. Rec.* **55**, 281–3.

—— (1980b). Economic appraisal—Thailand. *Weekly Epidemiol. Rec.* **55**, 289–92.

—— (1981). Economic appraisal—Indonesia. *Weekly Epidemiol. Rec.* **56**, 99–101.

Glassroth, J., Robins, A. G., and Snider, D. E. (1980). Tuberculosis in the 1980s. *New Engl. J. Med.* **302**, 1441–50.

Grab, B. and Cvejtanovic, B. (1977). Simple method for rough determination of the cost–benefit balance point of immunisation programmes. *Bull. Wld Hlth Org.* **45**, 536–41.

Grosse, R. N. (1980). Interrelation between health and population: observations derived from field experiences. *Social Sci. Med.* **14C**, 99–120.

Henderson, R. H. (1981). Letter to *Trans. R. Soc. Trop. Med. Hyg.* **75**.

Lancet (editorial) (1981). Rationalising measles vaccination. *Lancet* 236–7.

Litvinov, S., Assaad, F., Lundbeck, H., and Beausoleil, E. (1979). *Report on Ghana feasibility studies on immunisation* EPI/GEN/79/3. World Health Organization, Geneva.

Makinen, W. M. (1979). *A social cost-benefit analysis of anti-measles vaccinations in Yaoundé, Cameroon.* (PH.D dissertation) University of Michigan.

People's Democratic Republic of Yemen, *National Health Programme 1979–1983*, Aden.

Pönnighaus, J. M. (1979). *The cost-benefit of measles immunisation: a study from southern Zambia.* Medizin in Entwicklungslandern, Vol. 3, Peter Lang, Frankfurt-am-Main.

Stilwell, J. (1976). Benefits and costs of the schools' BCG Vaccination Programme. *Br. med. J.* **1**, 1002–4.

Walsh, J. A. and Warren, K. S. (1979). Selective primary health care: an interim strategy for disease control in developing countries. *New Engl. J. Med.* **301**, 967–74.

WHO (World Health Organization) (1977). *EPI training manual.* World Health Organization, Geneva.

Author's note

The author would like to thank Dr R. H. Henderson and colleagues in the Expanded Programme on Immunization of the World Health Organization for their assistance in obtaining material and offering advice, whilst absolving them from any responsibility for remaining errors or personal opinions expressed in this chapter.

9

Economics and nutrition planning

Gill Westcott

Introduction

The aim of this chapter is to show how certain economic techniques and approaches can be useful in nutrition planning. Because it attempts to write for health economists about nutrition problems, and for nutrition and health planners about economics, readers from both backgrounds may find something familiar and something new.

The next section describes what nutrition planning is, and considers why and when nutrition planning is necessary. Following this there is a section which discusses ways of identifying and measuring the extent of malnutrition. This discussion is continued in the next section, which explores the causes of malnutrition. Some alternative approaches to the analysis of nutrition problems are described, including the application of the economic concepts of demand and supply functions. This process of problem definition is an essential pre-requisite to the choice of strategies and programmes to tackle nutrition problems. The final section describes how techniques of economic evaluation can contribute to the choice of appropriate nutrition projects and to the inclusion of nutrition objectives in the evaluation of projects in other sectors.

As in the planning of any other health-related activities, particular problems are raised in the sphere of nutrition by the difficulties in measuring programme impact; the intangibility and yet the obvious importance of some of the benefits; and by the multiplicity of factors which impinge on nutritional status and which have to be taken into account when designing projects. It is argued that some of the techniques described below will facilitate the use of information in making planning decisions.

Nutrition planning

Nutrition planning may be simply defined as planning for nutrition objectives. This leaves open such questions as how the objectives of such planning can be precisely specified, and what instruments may be considered. These questions receive full discussion in Joy (1978*a*). Like all planning, nutrition planning is concerned with collective action (as opposed to individual action); but it need not always be undertaken by central government. The preparation of collective actions, the consideration of alternative approaches, and the policy decisions which are implied in that process, may be done at regional or local level, by sections of local government or within the Ministry of Health, or even within particular hospitals, clinics, or centres of health services.

A conventional description of formal planning activities would include the following processes (WHO 1979; Schofield 1979; Berg 1973):

— setting overall policies;
— problem definition and analysis;
— identification of alternative programmes;
— costing and evaluation of alternatives, leading to programme choice;
— implementation;
— evaluation.

This chapter, therefore, considers the contribution of economics to these processes as they relate to nutrition planning, assuming that the overall development policies have already been defined by central government.

There is often a tendency among health planners to assume that nutrition programmes are those aspects of the health services which are specifically directed to nutrition, such as nutrition education activities and the distribution of foodstuffs within under-five clinics. In reality, nutritional status, like health status, is affected by a wide range of government policies: agricultural development; food prices and wage levels; employment opportunities; distribution systems; sanitation; school feeding; and the education and role of women, for example.

Opinions differ, however, about whether nutrition planning should embrace all these factors. In effect, this would mean that the projects and policies of all Ministries would be scrutinized for their likely impact on nutrition, either by those responsible for programme evaluation within each of the departments and Ministries (as recommended by the World Bank (1974)), so that the impact on nutritional status would be added to the criteria for programme choice; or by the setting up of a Nutrition Planning Unit whose job it would be to examine programmes passed to it from other Ministries and to evaluate their implications for nutrition (Joy and Payne 1975).

This view is called the 'intellectual establishment view' by Field (1977), and criticized thus: 'In seeking to harness a total system behind rather limited goals it runs the risk of accomplishing very little.' He argues that no particular Ministry has an interest in the success of multisectoral activities, but rather in increasing the budget allotted to its own sphere of activities. Therefore multisectoral nutrition planning is unlikely to be successful. What he calls the 'bureaucratic view' of nutrition planning, namely that it is limited to specific nutrition-related *activities* such as school feeding, nutrition education, etc., is more likely to represent the realistic scope of nutrition planning in most countries, even though it concentrates on process and often fails to analyse strategy.

A more extensive criticism can also be made of nutrition planning as a whole: it might be argued that since the incidence and prevalence of malnutrition is so strongly related to low income, the adoption of a development policy which gives priority to raising low incomes and providing for basic needs will auto-matically bring about improvements in nutrition. This argument implies that there is no need for a separate nutrition policy. On the other hand it can also be argued that in circumstances where specifically egalitarian policies are not adopted, there is little chance for effective nutrition planning. If it is accepted that in developing countries the main nutritional objective is to reduce mal-nutrition, and since those who suffer from malnutrition are likely to be worst off financially, and since the distribution of food tends also to correspond to the distribution of power in the country, one may be sceptical about the possibility of changing one without the other. In both cases, it could be con-cluded that nutrition planning is either pointless or ineffective.

However, even in countries whose governments are committed to basic needs or redistributional approaches, reduction of poverty is not a short-term strategy. In the meanwhile, it may be possible to reduce some of the worst effects of malnutrition by policies related specifically to nutritional objectives. Moreover, not all nutritional problems are the result of poverty. There may be groups whose nutritional needs are more specific and can be met by suitably designed programmes (for instance the addition of Vitamin A to flour or meal is a relatively cheap measure and can prevent blindness). Therefore, it may be fruit-ful to plan measures such as these irrespective of whether or not a commitment to reduce poverty exists; and beyond this rather narrow scope, a wide range of policies can usefully be included in nutrition planning where governments are able to mobilize and redistribute resources and can achieve intersectoral co-ordination.

Definition and measurement problems

The identification of malnutrition in individuals and its measurement as a social problem does not necessarily require economic insights. However, it is an essen-tial area in planning and the economist must be aware of the conceptual and methodological issues involved.

Some nutritional problems in individuals can be clinically identified. Table 9.1 lists some of the major nutritional disorders. However, for every child in the developing world with overt clinical malnutrition there are many who have insufficient food to grow anywhere near as fast or as large as their genetic potential would allow. Lack of growth or slow growth is often associated with permanent physical and even mental damage (Church 1977; Leitzmann 1977*a*). It is associated with reduced resistance to infection (Leitzmann 1977*b*), increased mortality (Wittmann, Moodie, Fellingham, and Hausen 1967), and retarded school performance (Coovadia, Adhikari, and Mthethwa 1975; Popkin and Lim-Ybanez 1982). Inadequate growth, therefore, is a real problem for health and for national development, even when it does not result in clinically apparent illness.

Inadequate growth can be identified by anthropometric (body) measure-ments. One method is to plot the weights of well-nourished children against their

TABLE 9.1. *Clinically identifiable nutritional disorders*

Name	Symptoms	Deficiency	Source of nutrient
Kwashiorkor	Large belly, light thin hair, oedema (swelling); extreme cases have skin lesions	Protein/energy*	
Marasmus	Very thin	Protein/energy	
Pellagra	Dark skin on neck and arms, diarrhoea	Nicotinic acid (Niacin)	Groundnuts
Vitamin A deficiency	Night blindness; eventually, total blindness	Vitamin A	Fruit, vegetables, fish
Scurvy	Gums swell and bleed, loss of teeth, broken blood-vessels	Vitamin C	Fruit, green vegetables
Rickets	Aching joints, bones bend	Vitamin D	Sunlight, eggs, milk, fish, liver
Anaemia	Weakness, tiredness, thin blood	Iron	Green vegetables, legumes
Goitre	Swelling in neck	Iodine	Often in water
Obesity	Overweight, high blood pressure	Excess	

*Protein is used up by the body as energy when calorie intakes are very low. Therefore in most malnourished groups, supplementary energy intake will also provide enough protein for the body's requirements (Sukhatme 1972; Joy 1973).
Source: King *et al.* 1972.

age, and to use this as a standard against which other children can be assessed. In some areas the Harvard Standards (devised by using well-nourished Boston children) are accepted as representing the true genetic potential of children. In some areas local standards have been developed. Lines are plotted on a graph showing the average weight for age and (say) the third percentile (that line below which only three per cent of the well-nourished children fall). The third percentile is sometimes taken as the lower limit for well-nourished children, so that in a population where food deficiency is prevalent, any child falling below the third percentile can be considered malnourished. Another method frequently used is the Goméz Classification (Goméz, Ramos-Galvan, Frenk, Cravioto, Chavez, and Vazquez 1956) which also classifies children by weight for age. Less than 90 per cent of the standard is regarded as 'first degree malnutrition', less than 75 per cent as 'second degree' and less than 60 per cent as 'third degree malnutrition'; however, the use of this standard has been much criticized (Mata 1978).

For regular growth monitoring, the weight or the height of children for their age is preferred. However, in surveys to screen for nutritional problems some authorities prefer to use weight for height as a standard (Mata 1978; Walker and Richardson 1973). This implies that even if children are small for their age they are considered adequately nourished if they are not too thin for their height. However, this assumption is also the subject of fierce debate, and the appropriate criterion can only be determined by looking at how children who are exceptionally small but have adequate weight for height progress in their general health, at school, and in later life.

Use is frequently made of the Waterlow classification (Waterlow 1972) which divides children into four classes by weight-for-height and height-for-age. The virtue of this method is that it distinguishes chronically malnourished children (stunted) from the acutely malnourished (wasted). Head circumference, mid-upper-arm circumference, and skinfold thickness can also be used to identify nutritional status. The arm circumference measure is a convenient one for rapidly screening a large population of children for malnutrition because it is quick and uses very little equipment. The mid-upper-arm circumference changes so little between the ages of one and five years that measurements by means of a piece of string or X-ray tape with the critical dimensions marked on it (The Shakir Strip) can be used to screen large numbers of children for malnutrition without knowing their exact ages (Shakir and Morley 1974). Although a very stringent test, and one which misses oedematous children, it can be useful for comparing populations.

The causes of malnutrition

In addition to the well recognized problems in defining and measuring malnutrition, it is clear that there are a wide range of factors which influence food consumption and which must be borne in mind when looking for the causes of nutrition problems. Table 9.2 indicates some of the different kinds of problems which may give rise to nutritional deficiency. It also indicates how strategies to cope with the deficiency follow from an identification of its causes. A key question to ask is this: 'Is there any time of the year when families lack food?' If the answer is 'yes', the table shows that a constraint exists on food consumption arising from inadequate production, storage, or distribution systems, or from inadequate household purchasing power. If the answer is 'no', then the table indicates that problems of ignorance, food preparation, or food distribution within the family are responsible, and educational measures alone may be sufficient to improve matters.

The scheme in Table 9.2 can be used to arrive at a preliminary 'community diagnosis' of nutrition problems. It is suggested that a few community leaders (such as chiefs, shopkeepers, schoolteachers, health workers) *and* a sample of consumers be asked about all these possible causes of malnutrition (Brown and Brown 1979). In this way a list of appropriate interventions can be drawn up for consideration in the design of programmes. If there is to be a survey of nutritional problems it can be better designed after this preliminary investigation. However, this method can only be successful in a small, homogeneous community, where the causes of malnutrition are similar for everyone. At

TABLE 9.2. *Some causes of malnutrition*

	YES — Matters where education by itself cannot help			DOES FAMILY LACK FOOD AT ANY TIME IN THE YEAR?		NO — Matters where health and nutrition education can help, even alone
	Production →	Storage →	Transport/ marketing →	Purchasing →	Choice of food →	Preparing/cooking→eating/digesting dividing in family
Problems	Too little produced Seasonal shortages	Food rots, eaten by vermin etc.	Food doesn't reach market in remote areas Hoarding High mark-ups (shops in poor areas especially)	Can't afford enough food (especially artificial infant food) or enough variety	Mother unaware of nutritional needs (e.g. gives refined porridge only as weaning food) Infant food too bulky for child to get enough nutrients	Bottle-feeding – feed too diluted, bottle unhygienic Vitamins boiled out Protein thrown away (e.g. bean water) Children not given nutritious food e.g. eggs Small children get less — Child infected; no appetite or doesn't digest food (e.g. worms)

Underlying factors	Small land-holdings High rents Seasonal drought Poor agricultural know-how Lack of capital, labour, equipment	Storage techniques and customs	Poor rural communications Traders' monopolies Many middle-men	Low income (may be due to low production or wages) Income poorly managed Income not shared by wage-earner with family	Low weaning age Breakdown of traditional food habits Advertising	Lack of knowledge Habits, e.g. all eat out of one bowl Children neglected at home while mother works	Water supply Sanitation Knowledge of hygiene Unplanned urban settlement can accentuate these problems
Policy	Agricultural policy: does it give small farmers a chance? Does it give them access to inputs? Irrigation Land reform Supplement farm incomes by selling handmade goods; or rural industries (food processing, etc.)	Better storage: (a) at home (b) in bulk	Better transport Marketing co-operatives Buying co-operatives Marketing Boards	Wage levels Employment (see production) Food distribution (e.g. milk for kwashiorkor) Food vouchers Food subsidies Social security payments Family planning services New foods	Nutrition education Fortified food (e.g. add Vitamin A to flour) Child spacing (helps breast-feeding)	Nutrition education, including cooking Hygiene education (e.g. cup and spoon method) Small children have own bowls Day care facilities for working mothers	Provision of water and sanitation (site and service for shanty towns) Hygiene education Immunization Easily available health services

a national level, the picture is more complex and information may need to be collected in a more systematic way.

Food balance sheets

One method which has been used to identify and predict nutritional problems on a national scale is the construction of food balance sheets (Government of India 1968). An estimate is made of the total supply of staple foodstuffs for the country or region in question, and these estimates are compared, *either* with some estimate of minimal nutritional requirements for the population, *or* with likely demands for food. The object is to see whether there is, or will be a 'food gap' in aggregate terms (see Table 9.3).

TABLE 9.3. *Method of compiling a food balance sheet*

Supply	Requirements
1. Production = (area cultivated + projected growth) × (average yield + projected growth)	1. Requirements for human consumption = average minimum daily intake of protein, calories, and other nutrients* × total population†
2. Imports	2. Amount used for seed
3. Stocks	3. Amount used for feeding animals
4. *less* losses in storage	4. Amount in industrial uses
	5. Exports
	6. Stocks

*Several staple foods would have to be included in the balance sheet, or several separate balance sheets constructed, to consider how these requirements could be filled.
†Requirements are generally calculated separately for adults and children, people doing heavy labour, pregnant and lactating mothers, etc.
Source: Reported in Joy 1978*b*.

Such a procedure may be considered lacking in three ways. First, it derives only an estimate of the overall 'deficiency' or surplus; it does not indicate directly the relationship between food supplies and malnutrition. There is nothing to show how food, once produced, is distributed, and to whom. Due to inequalities or inefficiencies in distribution, it is possible for considerable malnutrition to exist even when the balance sheet shows a surplus. Secondly, it is not policy-oriented: there is no indication of how the recommended changes in production can be brought about, or how the additional food can be got to those who are deemed to be most in 'need'. Thirdly, even if the 'human consumption' part of the table were to be estimated by predicting the likely demand for foodstuffs from groups at projected income levels, no details would exist of what happens when the two sides are unequal, or of the effects which price changes might then have on both requirements and supply. Additional difficulties involved in the concept of 'minimum food requirements' are described by McArthur (1964).

Modelling the demand and supply of food markets

A more policy-relevant approach would be to model the demand and supply functions for a number of important food markets so as to be able to predict how both demand and supply will respond to various policy options such as subsidies, marketing policies, credit for producers, etc. (Taylor, L. 1978). To carry out an analysis for a staple grain, such as rice, would require the following:

1. *Construction of demand functions for target groups.* Data on how much specified population groups will purchase when the price of rice varies can be used to derive the 'demand curve' (shown in Fig. 9.1(a)). Similar functions can be constructed to show the response of consumers to a change in their household income (Fig. 9.1(b)), or in the price of substitute foods such as wheat (Fig. 9.1(c)). This figure shows only aspects of an overall demand function for rice which may be expressed as follows: $D_r = f(P_r, P_w, \bar{Y})$, which means that the demand for rice (D_r) depends on (= f) the price of

(a) **Price demand curve**

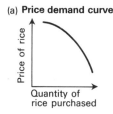

Shows price elasticity (responsiveness of demand to changes in price); prices of substitutes and incomes held constant

(b) **Income demand curve**

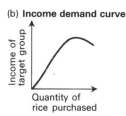

Shows income elasticity (responsiveness of demand to changes in incomes), with prices of rice, wheat, etc. given

(c) **Cross demand curve**

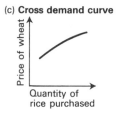

Shows cross-elasticity (responsiveness of rice purchases to changes in price of wheat), with price of rice and income levels given

Fig. 9.1. Aspects of the demand function for rice.

rice (P_r), the price of wheat (P_w), and some proxy figure such as an average or mode for incomes in the target community ($\overline{Y}$). Survey data will almost certainly be necessary to construct such a function for (say) the low income groups, and information from household expenditure surveys would be ideal for this purpose. Existing routine statistics are likely to cover the entire market demand and supply, not those of sub-groups.

2. *Construction of producers' supply functions.* A similar process can be carried out to model the way in which the food producers respond to factors such as the price which they can obtain for their crop, the prices of various inputs (seed, fertilizer, etc.), the availability of credit, and so on. For the cultivators, the higher the market price for their product the more they are likely to want to plant.

3. *Construction of the supply function to the market.* Because production of foodstuffs depends, among other things, on the market price, the amount *reaching* the market will also depend, broadly, upon the existing market price. However, it is also important to model aspects of the transport and distribution system which affect the quantities available after they leave the farm; these include losses in storage, costs of transport (supply to market may, for example, be reduced by a rise in oil prices), and the speculative behaviour of dealers who may withhold produce from the market if they believe that the price is about to rise. Such beliefs are hard to predict and very difficult to model. The likely shape of the supply curve to the market is shown in Fig. 9.2. This figure shows that the supply curve for rice is likely to be more price-elastic (responsive to price) in the long run than in the short run: a price rise may encourage a farmer to plant more rice and less wheat at the next planting; but if it continues it may become profitable for him to install irrigation facilities and cultivate two groups a year. Hence the supply curve will appear more like S^1S^1 if estimated over a long period of time.

These three systems, when modelled, may be helpful not only in discovering and explaining why some groups experience a shortage of food, but they can also be used to predict the effects of some policy interventions. Some examples appear later in this chapter, others are given in Joy (1978*a*). This kind of

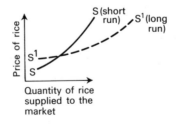

Fig. 9.2. The supply curve for rice.

information has also been used to analyse the impact of food aid. Large amounts of food surpluses have been given or sold to developing countries for soft currencies over the last three decades. About two-thirds of food aid is sold on the market by the receiving governments to increase supplies and generate funds for their projects. Unfortunately, this seems often to have depressed the domestic market price and reduced domestic agricultural production (Maxwell 1978). Only when food aid is distributed as food-for-work or to particular needy groups are these effects likely to be negligible (Stevens 1977).

A functional classification of malnutrition

It has been noted that the 'food balance sheet' approach has very limited scope in nutrition planning, and that a more detailed modelling of demand and supply relationships in foodstuffs, while illuminating, may be extremely costly in terms of data requirements and probably also computing expertise. As an alternative method for identifying and studying nutrition problems on a national or regional basis, Joy and Payne (1975) have proposed an approach which deals directly with nutritional status and can be done with less complicated data analysis. They recommend that an analysis should be made not only of the physiological types of malnutrition and the proximate causes (e.g. blindness in children caused by Vitamin A deficiency), but also of the types of population group who suffer from these conditions and why (e.g. children of migrant labourers who live in rural districts with low rainfall). This produces a 'functional classification' or dividing up of 'undernourished' populations into groups which have similar causes of nutrition problems and to which similar policies might be relevant. Table 9.4 gives an outline of such a functional classification, with divisions according to region, ecology, source of income, demographic categories, and deficiency patterns.

Joy and Payne suggest that this classification should precede extensive surveys of nutritional status. If a large-scale survey is done first, with an uninformed or arbitrary choice of categories, the sample size necessary to identify the types of malnutrition experienced will have to be unnecessarily large, thus increasing the cost of planning. Rather, they argue that the functional classification should be prepared first with the aid of available statistics. Then small surveys should be carried out in each group covered by the classification. In this way, a connection is made between food intake patterns and geographical location, income, and socioeconomic characteristics as well as with height/ weight data, morbidity, mortality, etc.

In conjunction with such a classification, Joy (1978a) follows an approach suggested by Berg and Muscat (1973) in suggesting the use of 'typical profiles' for each 'at risk' group of the population. These profiles, derived from studying in depth a few carefully chosen households, would describe the sources of food, methods of storage, amounts consumed, their nutritional value and constraints on the intake of nutrients, both outside the household (such as production, incomes, prices, availability) and inside the household (such as habits, customs,

TABLE 9.4. *Illustrative outline 'functional classification' of undernourished population as a basis for food and nutrition planning*

1. *Regional divisions*—based on administrative structure
2. *Ecological sub-zones*
      including, e.g. urban
                              rural accessible—irrigated; unirrigated
                              rural inaccessible—arable; grazing
      as well as subdivisions by cropping areas
3. *Economic status of sub-groups of population*
      including, e.g. urban—migrants recently arrived
                              —poor, stable employment: in large firms
                                                                       in small firms
                              —poor: unstable employment or unemployed
                              —income above subsistence
               rural—settled farmers—'surplus' farmers
                                              —'deficit' farmers
                      —nomads
4. *Demographic categories within sub-groups*
      including, e.g. mother–child (infants)
                              pre-school children
                              school-aged children
                              adults—male
                                           female
                              elderly
5. *Deficiency pattern*
      chronic
      seasonal
      occasional
6. *Nutrient deficiency (or problem)*

protein-calorie	calcium
vitamin A	iron
riboflavin	iodine
vitamin C	(lathirysm)

Source: Joy and Payne 1975.

and beliefs affecting the preparation and consumption of food). Such profiles provide a convenient format for gathering and presenting information in a way which will contribute to programme design and may help to ensure that the approaches chosen are acceptable and likely to be effective.

Economic evaluation of nutrition programmes

Evaluation may fulfil many purposes. The kind of evaluation or monitoring of nutrition programmes to ensure that they are being carried out according to plan, and that the correct activities are being performed, is generally one in which technical knowledge and managerial skill, rather than economic expertise, is brought to bear, though financial management is an important aspect of monitoring. It is in the *choice* of programmes where economic techniques of evaluation are most useful, whether the evaluation is done on the basis of estimates before a project proceeds or after its implementation.

The purpose of economic evaluation is to improve efficiency: that is, to achieve the maximum in terms of the chosen objectives with a minimum cost in resources. In choosing programmes, three types of comparison may be involved:

(1) between alternative nutrition programmes designed to accomplish the same objective;
(2) between nutrition and other programmes, to indicate whether the benefits of nutrition programmes justify resources being allocated to them; and
(3) between programmes whose implementation would have nutritional consequences which should be considered alongside their other costs and benefits.

The first type of comparison can be handled by cost-effectiveness analysis, provided that the objectives of the two programmes are identical and can be measured in the same terms (such as a reduction in the proportion of children underweight for their height). The second type of comparison, between nutrition and other projects, can in theory be handled by cost–benefit methodology. With the third type of comparison, it is essential that the choice of development programmes is not made in ignorance of the consequences for nutrition; this will merit at the least an examination of nutritional effects as part of the overall evaluation, whether or not this is undertaken within a cost–benefit framework.

Costing nutrition programmes

The costing of nutrition programmes is an essential component of evaluation and should be subject to the same considerations as costing exercises for any public project (see Chapters 7 and 8 for illustrations relating to health projects). These are that emphasis should be placed on:

(1) marginal costs—the addition to costs incurred by a programme rather than average (i.e. unit) costs; and
(2) social costs—the costs borne by society.

Private cost may be defined as the cost falling upon the individual recipient of goods or services provided, such as the fee or charge for a course of medicine. Budgetary cost is the cost falling on the government: in this case it might be the cost of providing the medicine, net of any contribution made by the patient in fees. However, in public programmes it is most appropriate to identify the 'social' costs and compare these to benefits in making decisions on resource allocation. The social cost is defined here as the sum of all costs involved in the provision of a good or service, whether they fall upon the recipient, the government, or other individuals, and whether they are in terms of money or not. Social costs are the benefits that society foregoes (opportunity cost) by having the good or service in question and not another good or service.

In a free market economy, the price of a resource is supposed to represent its value in the next best alternative use, and so is equal to its social cost.

However, for various reasons this is not always so. The divergences between market price and social cost are sometimes very obvious. For example, in a country with a controlled exchange rate, foreign exchange may be worth far more than the official market price. If some foreign currency has to be spent on imported foodstuffs, the actual cost in terms of its other uses, say replacing parts on industrial machinery, can be more than the nominal price would suggest. Thus, in costing projects, an adjusted price is sometimes used to estimate the true social cost: this is known as a 'shadow price'. It may not be the actual price the government has to pay, but it represents the value of the next best alternative foregone.

For the same reason, it is common for planning bodies in developing countries to use a shadow price for such as agricultural workers which is *lower* than the market wage rate. This is because, although an unskilled worker on a government agricultural programme has to be paid a wage in cash, the production foregone by that person, if he or she was previously unemployed, would be very low indeed; so little social product is lost by their employment on the public programme. Detailed methods of working out shadow prices are given in Dasgupta, Marglin, and Sen (1972), and further examples of their use have already been given in earlier chapters in this volume.

The criteria for cost-effectiveness

A programme is more cost-effective than another if it achieves the same objective with fewer resources, or if a given expenditure produces greater beneficial effects. This technique is the least ambitious of the various tests of efficiency, and is potentially a most useful instrument in the evaluation of nutrition programmes. None the less, it is crucial that the chosen measures of effectiveness are appropriate. Ideally, the programme cost should be related to any changes produced by the programme in the prevalence of malnutrition in the community, or perhaps to infant and child mortality. To do this, very carefully controlled field trials are required to distinguish the effects of nutrition programmes from those of other variables such as agricultural production, employment opportunities, and cultural and educational factors.

An example of such a study is that carried out at Narangwal Rural Health Research Centre, India, though it did not relate effectiveness to costs (Taylor, C. 1978). Similar groups of villages received different types of intervention to determine whether infection control alone, or a programme of nutritional education and supplementary feeding alone was more effective in reducing the prevalence of malnutrition and infant mortality. The finding that infection control was as effective as direct nutrition intervention in reducing mortality and malnutrition in children from two to three years, and more effective for children under two, provides essential information for the choice of more extensive programmes. The conclusion reached was that simply increasing food production would not have brought about significant improvements of health and nutrition; even in villages where a combined programme of nutrition and infection control was implemented and a reduction of 40 per cent in child mortality achieved, a hard core of malnourished children (mainly female) remained to whom the programme had made little difference.

Another study, in Jamaica, found that a programme of regular home visiting by rural women trained in short courses was able to reduce infant mortality by half within a year (Alderman and Levy 1973). It was concluded that the weighing alone of children was effective in this situation. Food was available, and once the mothers were aware of a problem they were able to remedy it.

Although these two studies did not proceed to carry out a full cost-effectiveness analysis, they do indicate the nature of the problems involved in undertaking the identification of the likely impact of nutrition programmes, and of each separate element within them, which is needed for informed policy-making. The importance of this point can be seen from the study of Berner (1977). He was able to report a reduction in the proportion of underweight children visiting Maternal Child Health clinics in Malawi from 40 per cent in 1970 to 23 per cent in 1976 following a programme of nutrition education, and regular weighing and feeding for malnourished children at clinics throughout the country. However, the supplementary food was provided free by the World Food Programme. It is not clear whether a large part of the reduction was due to these supplies, and a study of the cost-effectiveness of each part of the programme (with the food valued at the domestic cost) would help decide which parts to retain if the World Food Programme resources were withdrawn. Maxwell (1978) points out that since an estimated 95 per cent of all child nutrition programmes in developing countries involve supplementary feeding it is most unfortunate that few adequate estimates of their cost-effectiveness have been made. After surveying several studies he concludes that because externally provided food aid is often less acceptable to consumers, involves less community participation in feeding programmes, and because it may cause changes in tastes which are costly to maintain (such as use of dried milk), supplementary feeding programmes may not be a cost-effective use of food aid. He recommends the use of local foodstuffs where possible.

A quite different indicator of effectiveness was that used in Reutlinger and Selowsky's World Bank study (1976). Their measure of effectiveness was the amount of food purchased by the target population groups, and this was related to the budgetary cost of various interventions. They were able to show how the effects of general food price subsidies, income transfers, and selective subsidies (such as food stamps or vouchers) depended on the elasticity of demand for foodstuffs. Using the USA as an illustration, they calculated that a selective subsidy would cost the government about $1.33 for each extra dollar of food purchased by the groups at risk, compared with $5-18 for a general food subsidy, or $2 for an income subsidy. Not surprisingly, a general food subsidy would cost more because it would be given to everyone, not only to the target groups.

The value of this particular study, however, is limited by the narrow range of nutrition policies considered, by the inclusion of government costs only (not all social costs) and by the definition of benefits as extra food purchased, rather than a direct measure of the effects on nutrition. There should have been an estimate of how food purchases are related to nutritional status, and the assumption that selective subsidies will succeed in covering all the target population is probably unrealistic. However, the study illustrates a useful method for predicting some of the effects of some policies. A later work (Reutlinger and Alderman 1980) does predict the effect of income changes on the prevalence of deficient diets using information on income distribution, consumption and income elasticities.

A final problem common to all the studies so far mentioned is that whether the effectiveness was measured in terms of mortality, rates of malnutrition, or budget savings, only some of the benefits of the programme are captured in this manner. Programmes of infection control or small-scale food production, for example, can have extremely widespread effects and harmonize well with other developmental or health objectives. This complementarity cannot be counted in the cost-effectiveness methodology, though it can be dealt with by cost–benefit techniques. Most nutrition programmes, however, are chosen without even an estimate of the expected impact on nutritional status or general health. The provision of this kind of basic information alone would do much to improve the data available for decision-making.

Cost-benefit analysis of nutrition programmes

The cost–benefit framework is the natural one within which the various benefits of nutrition programmes, whether in the form of health, production, employment, or whatever, can be investigated. It involves estimating, as fully as possible, both the costs and benefits of programmes so that they can be compared with one another, and the ratio of costs to benefits can be compared with that achieved through other programmes.

The difficulties are both theoretical and practical. The beneficial effects of nutrition programmes may include not only increased productivity of workers in the short run—this will in fact be a minor part of the contribution to GNP if unemployment is prevalent—but also an improved ability to benefit from other social investments such as education, training, or agricultural extension and infrastructure. Moreover, by reducing infant and child mortality, successful nutrition programmes may in due course lead to a reduction in the birth rate and in the enormous investment of time, energy, and other resources in raising children who do not survive to adulthood. These benefits may be extremely long-term, and the relationships between nutrition and the returns on other investments are not well-mapped, even if the initial impact on nutritional status is known.

Some attempts have been made to calculate the contribution of nutrition programmes to GNP, on the grounds that the low priority given to such programmes has stemmed from a belief that they are 'unproductive'. Correa and

Cummins (1970), for example, estimate that increases in calorie consumption alone contributed to about five per cent of the growth of National Product of nine Latin American countries between 1950 and 1962, and a larger proportion of the growth in output per head. The econometric methods, however, are based on quite unrealistic assumptions about how the economy works, and no other justification is offered than that the results are 'useful'.

Though it is desirable to know all the effects of a programme, it is highly questionable whether the justification for nutrition programmes should depend solely or even mainly on their relationship to GNP (Joy 1973). True, the long-term increase in the basic necessities of life is a worthy goal of development, but GNP does not necessarily capture the nature of this goal. There are many benefits of nutrition programmes which, like the benefits of other development programmes, are not included in GNP calculations but can profoundly affect the quality of life or degree of suffering of populations. Some can be given a money value but others, despite various attempts, cannot be sensibly expressed in such terms. It follows that, if cost–benefit analysis includes only those 'quantifiable' benefits which *can* be expressed in money terms, its use as a single criterion to aid decision-making may result in the rejection of many nutrition programmes, even though they are desirable on health and welfare grounds.

Some of the difficulties with cost–benefit analysis stem from the unquestioning use of a 'cost' and 'price' structure determined by the distribution of income and wealth in a country; others from the way health benefits are valued by taking earnings as a proxy either for production or for 'worth' to society. Further, procedures to set values empirically upon intangibles such as pain and suffering have not yet proved very satisfactory. Likewise, imputing the 'value' of saving life, or limbs, or eyesight, from decisions made in practice will tend to reflect the actual high values placed (large expenses incurred) on some people's lives, and low values on others. The differences may reflect social inequality and the existing distribution of political power, or merely the fact that once the name of a suffering or endangered individual is known, vast amounts may be spent to save them (e.g. people lost at sea).

So the employment of a cost–benefit analysis to evaluate nutrition programmes, at least when a conclusive answer in terms of a rate of return is expected, may be a counsel of despair, if decisions were to be made on this kind of information. The conclusions of cost–benefit analysis are very rarely '*valid*' unless they use valuations on which some social consensus exists. In certain cases, of course, cost–benefit studies can yield conclusive results without there being a valuation problem. This occurs where a programme can be shown to yield monetary benefits to the government; and, where it is also known that all the other social effects, quantifiable or not, are beneficial. This is often the case with food fortification, which involves the adding of small amounts of 'missing' nutrients to staple foodstuffs. Many staple foods (e.g. flour) are processed on a large scale and, being very cheap to fortify, diminish considerably the number of malnourished requiring hospital services. In South Africa, for instance, it has been estimated that pellagra costs the health services over R2 million a year, and that after paying the programme cost, 70 per cent of this amount could be saved by supplementation of maize meal with niacin (SAMRC 1977).

Hence, the use of cost–benefit analysis as a process to identify and, where possible, measure all the relevant costs and benefits of programmes and so assist a considered discussion of the various issues involved can be extremely productive. The methodology can help policy-makers and at times the public to identify which values are crucial in a given decision and those which are not; and a continuous use over time may help to achieve greater consistency in programme choice. The fact that CBA may not give unambiguous conclusions on nutrition programmes does not mean that this method is particularly un-suited to use in the nutrition or health sector. For if it is unacceptable to deter-mine nutrition programmes on the basis of CBA, can it then be acceptable to choose, say, agricultural projects on this basis when they may have an equally profound impact upon levels of health and nutrition?

Economic evaluation of the nutritional impact of other programmes

Since, in any developing country, the determination of nutritional status is the outcome of many sectoral development policies, the best combinations of nutrition and other objectives (i.e. the most favourable trade-offs) can only be achieved by including nutritional objectives in the evaluation and choice of all programmes. Otherwise, there is a risk that one government ministry will be spending to achieve its own objectives, and the department concerned with nutrition will be spending more money simply to undo the unfavourable effects on nutrition (setting up a commercial beer industry might fall into this cate-gory). A harmonization of policies, therefore, could have advantages for the maximum achievement of a variety of objectives.

This harmonization can be attempted in two ways. The first is to ensure that any routine evaluation of public projects includes an investigation of their nutritional impact, and that this is given due weight in programme choice. Alternatively, relevant projects could be passed to a special Nutrition Planning Unit, which would use its own expertise to identify their impact on nutrition, and which would be charged with the responsibility of making recommenda-tions relevant to the acceptance or rejection of the programme or to its design. The possible nature and role of such a Nutrition Planning Unit is discussed in Joy and Payne (1975).

The possibilities for including consideration of the impact on nutrition within the routine evaluation frameworks of other programmes are consider-able; so, however, are the difficulties. Some of the relevant data for estimating the impact of development programmes on nutrition has to be obtained from the kind of surveys mentioned earlier. Only if the groups at risk from mal-nutrition have been identified, and the constraints on their intake of nutrients analysed, can these estimates be attempted. Likewise, for the reasons discussed above, valuation problems will arise if the nutritional impact is to be included within the framework of a cost-benefit study. For instance, one fundamental issue is whether the benefits are to be valued equally, irrespective of the nutritional or income levels of the beneficiaries. Many would argue that it is desirable to weight any benefits according to the group which benefits, with a higher value placed upon increments to the lowest income groups, or those which fall furthest below a certain nutritional standard. Such weights could be identified in conjunction with policy-makers, or by using the values implied in past decisions and presenting them to policy-makers for discussion. However, such a procedure is rarely carried out; not only is it cumbersome but it may also be impolitic to try to define the values placed on income to various groups. Vagueness, a fault for planners, may be a politician's virtue.

Yet there is great concern, for instance, at the failure of many agricultural development programmes to provide more food for the poor. The adoption of such a weighting procedure could have had a dramatic effect on some of the measures taken over the last two decades. Hernandez, Pérez Hidalgo, Hernandez, Madrigal, and Chavez (1974) evaluated the nutritional impact of an agricultural programme in a fertile region of Mexico, and the findings, typical of many areas of outstanding production increases, indicated that although the general agricultural and economic situation in the country had improved a great deal, and although the children with normal growth had increased in weight considerably, the proportion with second and third degree malnutrition (Gomez, Ramos-Galvan, Frenk, Cravioto, Chavez, and Vazquez 1956) was not significantly different in 1971 from that in 1958. In short, despite overall improvements in agriculture, the total numbers of malnourished had actually increased.

The programmes which were carried out in the Mexican community in the above study included infection control, agricultural improvement, extension services, and the encouragement of cash crops for export. These elements have formed a common strategy throughout the world, and it has too often been assumed that an increase in agricultural production will raise nutrition standards. Ironically, even if the great increase in production is in foodstuffs (as in many Green Revolution areas) it does not follow that the malnourished will consume them.

Other sectors may also affect nutrition. The development of manufacturing may increase urban incomes at the same time as it causes earlier weaning of children so that women can work. (Crèches might avert some of the adverse consequences.) School feeding programmes and nutrition education, sanitation programmes which reduce parasitic infection, the balance of economic output, hours of work, choice of technology, and employment policy, all these affect nutritional status and this impact deserves to be assessed.

In view of the difficulties already mentioned with cost-benefit analysis, however, there may be no ready way of making the nutritional changes resulting from such programmes commensurable with their other costs and benefits. None the less, in some cases, where the main constraints on nutrition levels is household purchasing power and the main impact of a programme on nutrition will be via incomes, it may be sufficient to complete an analysis weighting increments according to the socioeconomic groups which benefit. In other cases, such as a scheme to provide sanitation for squatter housing, the benefits of infection control on nutrition may be measured, but not easily valued in money terms. In the absence of well-defined methods of valuing national objectives (providing national parameters for planning), it ought still to be possible to identify likely changes in nutrition even if these cannot be quantified or valued precisely in money terms.

Summary and conclusions

Nutrition planning has a role in all developing countries undertaking programmes which explicitly or implicitly contain nutritional objectives. Analysis of nutritional problems within the country and evaluation of alternative interventions can help to improve the efficiency and effectiveness of these programmes. The achievement of better nutritional standards can also be greatly assisted by a harmonization of nutritional objectives with other national objectives in the overall design and evaluation of development programmes.

This chapter has argued that planning for nutritional objectives should include the following steps:

Step 1: Identification of groups which are likely to be malnourished, and the nature and extent of their nutritional deficiencies. Small surveys to find out what proportion of various population groups experience nutrition deficiencies and why, are more likely to be useful in policy terms than nationwide or regional surveys to identify the overall extent and nature of malnutrition. A 'functional classification' of 'at risk' groups can inform such surveys and make their results more useful.

Step 2: Establishing the major causes of malnutrition in each group, whether it be inadequate availability of food, or income, or of knowledge, or inappropriate utilization of food within the family. An economic analysis of the causes of malnutrition may be required, to focus upon demand and supply determinants.

Step 3: Design of programmes which could have a nutritional impact on the various 'at risk' groups, and the evaluation of alternative interventions. This will involve a careful assessment of the effect to be expected upon the rates of malnutrition in the 'at risk' groups, and a comparison of the costs and effects of alternative programmes. Projects which depend for their success upon behavioural relationships (such as household consumption responses to price and income changes) may require econometric modelling of the relationships. When choosing between alternative programmes with the same objective (e.g. allowing a target group to consume more food, or reducing rates of malnutrition among under-fives), cost-effectiveness analysis is appropriate, showing how a given sum of money can be most productively spent. When choosing between programmes with different objectives, whether within nutrition, or between nutrition and other projects, a cost-benefit framework may be helpful, particularly when assessing some of the far-reaching effects of improving nutrition. These effects will, however, be expressed in different forms and units of measurement, and it must be accepted that not all costs and benefits are capable of being valued in money terms. Indeed, extremely sensitive assumptions are involved in such valuations:

Nutrition planners need not be dismayed that they cannot produce cost–benefit ratios comparable with those for other projects. It may be that the ratios calculated for the other projects are wrong and do not correctly reflect national objectives, and the relevant course of action therefore is to question the pricing assumptions which are being used for all evaluations (Joy and Payne 1975).

Step 4: Examination of the nutritional effects likely to result from existing development programmes whose main objective is not nutritional improvement, and presentation of the findings at a stage relevant to decisions on these plans, and prior to their implementation.

Step 5: Proposals concerning the package of nutrition-oriented measures or projects to be adopted, together with an estimate of the likely impact of these on the rates of nutritional deficiency predicted, and procedures for monitoring this impact over time.

This is an ambitious programme. It will be seen that the success of the later stages is dependent on that of the earlier ones. This means that the definition of the problem is particularly crucial, without which it is unlikely that the other steps will have much impact. It involves the establishment of a data base, not necessarily comprehensive or very detailed in the first instance. Thus in establishing a capability for nutrition planning, these are the areas for preliminary work.

Two sets of specific techniques—the description or estimation of economic relationships relevant to the causation of nutrition problems, such as the determination of food prices, consumption patterns, and production; and the evaluation of proposed projects—are central to the steps detailed above and are matters where economic expertise can be applied. Beyond this, the basic analytical approach by which economists analyse decisions (that of maximizing outputs with given resource constraints) is a convenient formalization of what planners must do to maximize attainment of their nutritional objectives.

REFERENCES

Alderman, M. H., and Levy, B., Husted, I., and Ryan, S. (1973). A young child nutrition programme in rural Jamaica. *Lancet* 1166–9.
Berg, A. (1973). *The nutrition factor: its role in national development.* The Brookings Institution, Washington DC.
— and Muscat, R. (1973). Nutrition program planning: an approach. In

Nutrition, national development and planning (ed. A. Berg, N. S. Scrimshaw, and D. L. Call), pp. 248-74. MIT Press, Cambridge, Mass.

Berner, H. (1977). Prevention of malnutrition in Malawi. In *Nutrition in developing countries* (ed. R. Korte). Deutsche Gesellschaft für Technische Zusammenarbeit (GTZ), West Germany.

Brown, J. E. and Brown, R. C. (1979). *Finding the causes of child malnutrition.* Teagle and Little, USA.

Church, M. A. (1977). Nutrition and physical performance. In *Nutrition in developing countries* (ed. R. Korte). Deutsche Geseleschaft für Technische Zusammenarbeit (GTZ), West Germany.

Coovadia, H. M., Adhikari, M., and Mthethwa, D. (1975). Physical growth of black children in the Durban area. (Mimeo.) University of Natal, South Africa.

Correa, H. and Cummins, G. (1970). Contribution of nutrition to economic growth. *Am. J. clin. Nutr.* 23, 560-5.

Dasgupta, P., Marglin, S., and Sen, A. (1972). *Guidelines for project evaluation.* United Nations: Industrial Development Organization (UNIDO), Vienna.

Field, J. O. (1977). The soft underbelly of applied knowledge: conceptual and operational problems in nutrition planning. *Food Policy* 2, 228-39.

Gomez, F., Ramos-Galvan, R., Frenk, S., Cravioto, J., Chavez, R., and Vazquez, J. (1956). Mortality in second and third degree malnutrition. *J. trop. Paediat.* 2, 77.

Government of India (1968). Draft plan document. (Mimeo.) Ministry of Health, New Delhi. (Described in Joy 1978*b*).

Hernandez, M., Pérez Hidalgo, C., Hernandez, J. R,, Madrigal, H , and Chavez, A. (1974). Effect of economic growth on nutrition in a tropical community. *Ecol. Food Nutr.* 3, 283-91.

Joy, L. (1973). Food and nutrition planning. *Institute of Development Studies reprint 107.* Institute of Development Studies (IDS), Sussex.

— (1978*a*). The concept of nutrition planning. In *Nutrition planning: the state of the art* (ed. L. Joy), pp. 107-22. IPC Science and Technology Press, Guildford.

— (ed.) (1978*b*). *Nutrition planning: the state of the art.* IPC Science and Technology Press, Guildford.

— and Payne, P. (1975). Food and nutrition planning. Food and Agriculture Organization, Rome.

King, M., King, F., Morley, D., Burgess, L., and Burgess, A. (1972). *Nutrition for developing countries.* Oxford University Press, Nairobi.

Korte, R. (ed.) (1977). *Nutrition in developing countries.* Deutsche Gesellschaft für Technische Zusammenarbeit (GTZ), West Germany.

Leitzmann, C. (1977*a*). Nutrition and mental development. In *Nutrition in developing countries* (ed. R. Korte), pp. 71-7. GTZ, West Germany.

— (1977*b*). Nutrition and infection. In *Nutrition in developing countries* (ed. R. Korte), pp. 217-24. GTZ, West Germany.

McArthur, M. (1964). Some factors involved in estimating calorie requirements with special reference to persons engaged in agricultural labour in Asian countries. *J. R. Statistics Soc.* 44, 392-408.

Mata, L. (1978). The nature of the nutrition problem. In *Nutrition planning: the state of the art* (ed. L. Joy), pp. 91-9. IPC Science and Technology Press, Guildford.

Maxwell, S. (1978). Food aid for supplementary feeding programmes. *Food Policy*, 289-98.

Popkin, B. M. and Lim-Ybanez, M. (1982). Nutrition and school achievement. *Social Sci. Med.* **16**, 53–62.

Reutlinger, S. and Selowsky, M. (1976). Malnutrition and poverty. *World Bank staff occasional paper No. 23.* World Bank, New York.

— and Alderman, H. (1980). The prevalence of calorie deficient diets in developing countries. *World Bank staff working paper No. 374.* World Bank, New York.

SAMRC (South African Medical Research Council) Project Group (1977). Food fortification in South Africa. (Mimeo.) South African Medical Research Council.

Schofield, S. (1979). *Development and the problems of village nutrition.* Institute of Development Studies, Croom Helm, London.

Shakir, A. and Morley, D. (1974). Measuring malnutrition. *The Lancet* i, 758–9.

Stevens, C. (1977). Food aid: more sinned against than sinning? *ODI Rev.* 2.

Sukhatme, P. V. (1972). The present pattern of production and availability of foods in Asia. In Three papers on food and nutrition: the problem and the means of its solution. *IDS Communication No. 101.* Institute of Development Studies, Sussex.

Taylor, C. (1978). Sectoral approaches to food and nutrition policy analysis. In *Nutrition planning: the state of the art* (ed. L. Joy), pp. 28–35. IPC Science and Technology Press, Guildford.

Taylor, L. (1978). The determinants of nutritional status: what economic planners need to know. In *Nutrition planning: the state of the art* (ed. L. Joy), pp. 9–17. IPC Science and Technology Press, Guildford.

Walker, A. R. P. and Richardson, B. D. (1973). International and local growth standards. *Am. J. clin. Nutr.* 897–900.

Waterlow, J. C. (1972). Classification and definition of protein-calorie malnutrition. *Br. med. J.* **3**, 566.

WHO (World Health Organization) (1979). *Formulating strategies for health for all by the year 2000.* World Health Organization, Geneva.

Wittmann, W., Moodie, A. D., Fellingham, S. A., and Hausen, J. D. L. (1967). An evaluation of the relationship between nutritional status and infection by means of a field study. *S. Afr. Med. J.* **41**, 664–82.

World Bank (1974). *Environmental, health and human ecologic considerations in economic development projects.* World Bank, Washington DC.

10

Health sector planning and national development planning

Mark Wheeler

Introduction

A decade ago Feldstein justly observed that, despite the contribution health improvements could make to the overall process of economic development, economists had generally remained silent on the subject of programmes of health care in developing countries and had made no attempt to extend the methods of economic optimization to the health care sector (Feldstein 1970). Likewise, public health administrators had not developed any systematic methods of planning or sought to integrate health care into the broader context of development planning. Today, notwithstanding the increasing interest which economists are displaying in the health sector—an interest gradually extending to developing countries—it remains a valid observation that planning for the health sector in developing countries retains its enclave character. The central planning authorities have failed to build into their models the acknowledged interactive relationships between the health sector and other sectors, and have failed to recognize these relationships in making resource allocations to health. Nor have the health authorities been able to elucidate the production function for health, or to specify the contribution of health to the social welfare function in a manner that convincingly substantiates their claims for more resources. The outcome of this mutual incomprehension is that, in the great majority of cases, planning for the health sector is an independent exercise in sub-optimization, carried out by health sector professionals within resource constraints defined in an essentially arbitrary manner by central economic planners.

Three facets of this situation will be explored in this chapter. First, the characteristics of the macroeconomic models underlying national development plans will be discussed, and it will be suggested that these models are not well adapted to incorporate the significant relationships of the health sector. Secondly, the current practice of national development planning will be reviewed, based on an analysis of a non-random sample of recent published plans. With few exceptions, these plans provide ample evidence to support the assertion that the health sector is planned largely independently of the overall national plan. Thirdly, different approaches to health sector planning will be considered, to investigate their methodologies and their relevance to developing country circumstances.

Macroeconomic planning models and the health sector

Although published development plans seldom reveal the method of their construction, Todaro has observed that there is a heavy reliance on the use of theoretical economic models:

In most poor countries, these models often form either the analytic base or the actual operational framework within which the detailed components of the development plan derive their specific quantitive values (Todaro 1971).

The models most frequently used are derivatives of the Harrod–Domar growth model; in a few countries, where the planning machinery is more sophisticated and the industrial structure more highly integrated, inter-industry models may also be used.

The key equation of the Harrod–Domar model can be written:

$$g = \frac{s}{k}$$

where g = the rate of growth of national income;
      s = the propensity to save;
      k = the incremental capital/output ratio.

Use of the Harrod–Domar model presupposes shortage of capital investment to be the primary economic constraint. Todaro, for example, comments:

The model is greatly simplified in the sense that savings, investment and income are the only variables considered, the implicit assumption being that limited supplies of high level manpower, fluctuations in the value of foreign aid, etc., are less crucial and that capital accumulation constitutes the central process by which all other aspects of development policy are made possible.

The model can be used either to predict the feasible rate of income growth, g, in the light of ascertained values for s and k, or to estimate the values of s and k required to satisfy an exogenously given target rate of income growth. Actual values can be altered by economic policies. The value of the parameter k may be reduced by improved methods of production or by varying the composition of investments. The value of the parameter s may be raised by efforts to stimulate private savings (personal and business) or by increased government savings (through taxation). In the absence of sufficient domestic savings, the government may seek foreign savings. Although the primary focus is on the rate of savings and investment, the model can be extended to deal with the implications for public revenue and the balance of payments of alternative growth rates by the addition of parameters representing tax rates and the propensity to import.

The model is of little operational value in this highly aggregate form. However, it can be elaborated into semi-aggregate two-sector or three-sector forms, where the sectors might be defined as investment goods and consumption goods industries, or export-oriented industries and domestic industries. Alternatively, the economy might be disaggregated into a greater number of broadly defined industrial sectors; for example, a projection model used in East Africa employed the six sectors of agriculture, manufactures, construction, transport, services, and government (Clark 1965). While these so-called main or leading sector models are an improvement on either the simple aggregate or semi-aggregate models, they are still highly abstract representations of the real economy:

> The two distinguishing characteristics of these models which make them so amenable to development planning . . . are, first, the relative simplicity of their construction and the ease of their mathematical manipulation and, second, the adaptability to the often crude and incomplete statistical information available in most poor countries. Their main drawbacks, however, lie in the rather sweeping nature of their economic generalisations, their failure to provide a detailed structural breakdown of the economy and their inability to ascertain whether or not a particular programme will result in an optimum allocation of available material, financial and human resources (Todaro 1971).

No inferences concerning the health sector can be drawn from models of this type. This is not necessarily a criticism of the models; after all, they were designed to demonstrate relationships of the macro-economy, and do not aim to provide detailed prescriptions for individual sectors, especially a sector such as health considered so relatively small and inert. There are several reasons for the failure of these models to give any guidance in planning the health sector. First, the models deal with the growth of income as measured by the national accounts, rather than the growth of welfare. The health services' contribution to the ultimate goal of enhanced welfare is likely to be relatively greater than their contribution to the proximate goal of increased income, because the national income accounting conventions fail to capture the full value of health services output. In the private sector, prices are distorted by multiple sources of market failure and in the public sector, health services are generally valued at the cost of resource inputs.

Secondly, the models implicitly treat the accumulation of physical capital as the sole source of growth of output and income. While the notion of 'human' capital could in principle be incorporated in the models, either by the addition of a parameter representing the stock of human capital, or by modification of the value of k to reflect the greater efficiency of physical capital when employed in conjunction with additional human capital, in practice capital accumulation is taken to refer to investment in buildings and equipment. A change in the health status of the labour force therefore remains unrecognized in the operation of these models, implying there is no need to invest resources in the health sector to bring about such a change.

Thirdly, in models of this type, the sectors into which the national economy is divided are so broad that the health sector cannot be separately distinguished. Depending on definitions, it will usually form part either of the services sector or of the government sector (and may sometimes be split between the two). Given that multisectoral models rarely employ more than ten sectors and that health typically accounts for only one or two per cent of national income in poor countries, it is hardly surprising that health is not separately identified. However, any overall estimates of demand, and implied capital investment, made for these broadly defined sectors do not necessarily apply to their health component. For instance, estimates of demand for government services are effectively determined by government policy decisions, and are not the product of spontaneous consumer demand. While the models may assume that government services will grow *pro rata* with national income, or grow more or less quickly according to stated government policies (Tinbergen 1967), there is clearly a potential conflict between the use of additional public revenues to expand services and their use to increase the capital stock in agriculture and manufacturing. As other chapters in this volume have also made plain (see especially Chapter 2), national planners may well wish to propose restraint in the expansion of services (assumed to meet only current consumption needs) in order to permit greater investment (assumed to expand the capacity to meet future consumption needs).

Fourthly, the treatment of the capital/output ratio in the models assumes that after an initial investment outlay there will be an associated constant annual output in all subsequent time periods. This mechanistic assumption does not closely accord with the experience of outlays in the health sector, where there is frequently a long gestation period between the initial outlay (whether funded from the capital or recurrent budget) and the moment when benefits are realized.

Fifthly, the models are extremely crude in the pattern of relationships they assume between variables. Typically, one variable is related to another by a single coefficient, assumed constant over time, such as the incremental capital/ output ratio which relates investment in one time period to incremental output in subsequent periods. The crudity and rigidity of these assumed relationships contrast with the now general understanding of the synergistic interaction of social forces and the multiple determinants of health status (Taylor and Hall 1967; Frederiksen 1969; WHO 1973; Grosse 1980). The relationships between health service activities and health status, as considered in some detail in Chapter 2, are mediated by a host of environmental and behavioural factors, which are in turn influenced by almost every aspect of the social and natural systems. Many of the benefits of better health derive from long-term demographic change; for example, gains in infant and child survival contribute to the adoption of the small family norm, which not only generates a demographic structure which is a more efficient factor of production, with lower dependency ratios and longer average duration of working life, but also produces further reductions in morbidity and mortality as the hazards of birth and early childhood are encountered relatively less frequently. Macroeconomic models are typically used for short- to medium-term projections, such as a five-year plan period within which demographic rates may reasonably be assumed to be constant. They therefore fail to reflect the cumulative effect of secular change which can ultimately be revolutionary in its impact.

Finally, since these macro models yield no prescriptions for the health sector as a whole, it is evident that they can provide no guidance on allocations within the health sector. Indeed, given the emphasis which they place on fixed capital investment, they may contribute to a climate of uncritical thought in which the health sector is urged to sacrifice growth of recurrent expenditure in order to finance expansion of the stock of buildings and equipment, notwithstanding the frequently glaring signs that the chief deficiencies in service stem from the shortage or absence of trained staff and lack of money for drugs and consumables, transport operating costs and equipment maintenance and repair, all of which are charges against the recurrent rather than the capital budget.

Inter-industry models represent a higher order of sophistication than leading sector models, with correspondingly large data requirements, but they provide very little further assistance to planners of the health sector. At the core of the inter-industry model is the input–output matrix which reveals the extent to which the output of each industry is dependent on purchases from other industries, from imports and from primary factors. The number of sectors distinguished in models of this type is highly variable and may run up to one hundred or more; the health services sector can be separately identified (although it is often amalgamated with other public services, since the degree of disaggregation of sectors tends to be very much greater for manufactures than for services). Even where there is a separate row and column vector for health services in the inter-industry matrix, this type of model still does not fully capture the interactive relationships of the health sector with other sectors. The principal reason is that the matrix is concerned with inter-industry purchases, whereas the health inputs to other sectors are not directly purchased by firms in those sectors but by their labour force, and consequently appear as final demand. Because of the apparent absence of inter-industry transactions, the expansion of other sectors of the economy implies no corresponding increase in the output of health services.

The main value of the inter-industry model is to provide a consistency check on the projected output of different sectors; an expansion of agricultural output, for example, is assumed to be dependent on an expansion of those industries supplying inputs to agriculture, such as fertilizers and transport. Unless an appropriate expansion is planned for these industries, the planned expansion of agriculture is likely to be thwarted. In conjunction with a model predicting the composition of final demand, the inter-industry model can also be used to estimate the additional inputs of labour and capital required for the planned expansion of output. In this way, the model provides the basis for allocating investment funds between sectors, and also gives some indication of the likely labour market demand for the output of the education sector. However, since the relationships between health and the labour supply are much more complex and diffuse, the implications for the output of health services are much less obvious.

As all output is assumed to be absorbed as final demand, the inter-industry matrix itself contributes nothing to the estimate of future output. As noted already, there are problems in forecasting the demand for public services (including health services), a common assumption being that the output of public services will grow *pro rata* with the economy in general. Tinbergen (1967) gave this assumption the title of 'the method of complementarity':

If the input–output method is applied in its most primitive form, it is assumed that all these activities take place in proportion to the national income or the income of certain sectors or regions. If the subject is approached in a rather more precise way, there is no need to assume that the social activities take place in proportion to income, but that the increases in the social services are proportional to increases in income.

It can be concluded that the only prescription from macroeconomic modelling for projecting allocations to the health sector is a casual recommendation to apply a simple averaging procedure, as is appropriate for minor residual items in any projection exercise. Such a procedure is less than ideal when applied to the health sector.

The only style of development planning in which prescriptions for the health sector are likely to derive from the central strategic calculations is the basic needs approach. This approach stems from a concern to provide people, especially the poorest, with their 'basic needs'. What basic needs comprise varies widely, from minimal requirements for survival, such as food, shelter, clothing, and health services, to psychological needs such as participation and democracy. The approach is not therefore an economic or social theory, but rather a movement directed at a series of priorities for action, which usually includes action on health. While the satisfaction of basic needs is one element in the economic policy and planning of a handful of countries, mainly in South Asia, nowhere is it the dominant inspiration for the allocation of resources, and, as yet, the methodology of basic needs determination is so elastic that each application is entirely idiosyncratic. Since this chapter concentrates on planning models of broad relevance actually in use, not on general ideologies of development, the basic needs approach is left to one side. It represents, however, an approach with some potential if it can be developed from a shopping list of requirements to a methodology for planning.

The current practice of national health planning

The practice of health sector planning in developing countries is explored below by reviewing thirty recent development plans (see Table 10.1). The set of plans examined were those published in English since 1970 and available to the author. While the set is not comprehensive, or the selection a random sample, the plans do embrace a considerable range of content and method.

TABLE 10.1. *List of development plans*

Country	Title of document	Plan period	Duration (years)	Underlying economic model
Bangladesh	The first five year plan	1973–1978	5	Leading sectors
Belize	Development plan	1977–1979	3	Public investment
Botswana	National development plan	1979–1985	5	Leading sectors
Ethiopia	Strategy outline for the fourth five year plan	1974/5 to 1978/9	5	Semi-aggregate
Fiji	Eighth development plan	1981–1985	5	Inter-industry
Ghana	Five year development plan	1975/6–1979/80	5	Inter-industry
Guyana	Draft second development plan	1972–1976	5	Aggregate
India	Draft sixth five year plan revised	1978–1983	5	Inter-industry
Indonesia	Third five year development plan (English summary)	1979–1984	5	Leading sectors
Iran	Fifth development plan revised	1973–1978	5	Leading sectors
Jamaica	Five year development plan	1978–1982	5	Aggregate
Jordan	Five year plan	1976–1980	5	Leading sectors
Kenya	Development plan	1970–1974	5	Leading sectors
Korea	Third five year economic development plan	1972–1976	5	Leading sectors
Lesotho	Second five year development plan	1975–1979/80	5	Leading sectors
Malaysia	Third Malaysia plan	1976–1980	5	Leading sectors
Mauritius	Five year plan for economic and social development	1975–1980	5	Leading sectors
Nepal	The fifth plan in brief	1975–1980	5	Leading sectors
Pakistan	Fifth five year plan	1978–1983	5	Leading sectors
Papua New Guinea	National public expenditure plan	1981–1984	3	Public investment
Philippines	Five year Philippine development plan	1978–1982	5	Leading sectors
Saudi Arabia	Second development plan	1975–1980	5	Leading sectors
Seychelles	National development plan	1978–1982	5	Public investment
Sierra Leone	National development plan	1974/5–1978/9	5	Leading sectors
Sri Lanka	The five year plan	1972–1976	5	Semi-aggregate
Sudan	The six year plan of economic and social development	1977/8–1982/3	6	Leading sectors
Thailand	Fourth national economic and social development plan	1977–1981	5	Leading sectors
Turkey	A summary of the third five year development plan	1973–1977	5	Inter-industry
Zambia	Second national development plan	1972–1976	5	Leading sectors

From studying the table, it can be seen that the most common type of macro-economic model underlying the national development plans was a leading sector(s) projection model. Only four plans achieved a higher level of sophistication, using an inter-industry matrix as a consistency check on sectoral production targets. The remaining three plans were evidently not based on any formal macroeconomic model, being simply compilations of capital expenditure proposals for the public sector, and were in effect 'public investment' plans.

As might have been predicted from the analysis of macroeconomic models, very few of the development plans included the health sector in the introductory sections or in discussions of overall development strategy, except in the context of a concern about rapid population growth. In 21 out of the 30 plan documents, excessive population growth was identified as an impediment to the growth of welfare; in most cases, the development of health services was favoured as part of the public policy response, recognizing either the potential contribution of health services to family planning programmes, or the impact of reduced infant and child mortality on fertility behaviour, or both interactions.

It is clear from studying the development plans that changes in the health status of the population were not treated as critical variables, though it is perhaps necessary to distinguish here between the introductory or strategy chapters of the plan document, and the health chapters themselves. The former are drafted by the macro-planners and reveal their preoccupations; the latter are drafted by the Ministry of Health and often have the tone of unconvincing apologias for expenditure on health services. In only five of the plans have the macro-planners acknowledged the positive impact of better health on labour productivity; in a further three cases the health planners have made the same point. The macro-planners are much more ready to acknowledge the contribution of health services to meeting distributional objectives and to the direct satisfaction of welfare needs; references appear in upwards of one-third of the plan documents. For instance, the First Five-Year Plan of Bangladesh states:

Investment in industry necessitates related investment in the power and transportation sector as well as in trade and ancillary services. Investment in the social sectors, such as health, education and family planning was determined primarily by the need to meet postulated social objectives.

and in a similar vein, the Second Lesotho Five-Year Development Plan states:

To promote social justice, the Plan proposes . . . a substantial improvement in the quality of health care and other social services.

The range and scope of activities included in the health sectoral plans differed widely from one country to another. In five cases, they were confined to the actions of the medical services; in only nine cases were they reasonably comprehensive, in that they embraced medical services, nutrition, family planning, water supply, and sanitation. At least half the plans confined their attention to Government health services and either made no mention of non-Government agencies or, in a few instances, acknowledged their existence but envisaged no action by them in the plan period. Specific references to the private health sector appeared in only one-third of the plans and none of them provided detailed forecasts of expenditures by non-Government agencies. In this connection, it is worth giving an extended quotation from India's Sixth Five-Year Plan (Revised Draft):

Health cannot be viewed in isolation from the overall goals and policies of national development; it is both an important input as well as a desirable end-product. Although rapid and equitable economic development is itself the best health care for the people, outlay on health has also to be accepted as investment in human capital which qualitatively contributes to economic development. For purposes of Plan allocation, outlay on health is confined to the health services sector programme of the Government, but for overall planning of health, other related programmes have to be taken into account, without which [the] health sector would remain deficient or would not be able to build the defence mechanism of the society against disease.

One slightly surprising finding was that there was no consistent relationship between the degree of sophistication of the macroeconomic plan and the comprehensiveness of the health sectoral plan. Two of the countries with plans based upon inter-industry models (Ghana and Turkey) revealed health sector plans with the narrowest scope. Conversely, several countries with distinctly crude macroeconomic plans (among them Papua New Guinea, Seychelles, and Indonesia, the latter explicitly denying that its plan was based upon a formal model) have health sector plans that are not only comprehensive in scope, but also explicitly recognize the complex determination of health status and envisage inter-sectoral action programmes to advance health.

The form in which health sector objectives were expressed in these plans was highly variable. In some cases, no clear statement of health objectives could be found and the principal objectives could only be inferred from the general drift of descriptive remarks. The most common form of objective, found in half the plans, was the expansion or improvement of health services, without direct reference to any higher order purpose (i.e. to the improvement of health itself). Yet nearly a third of the plans did state their objective to be an improvement in the health status of the population, while in a fifth of the plans an improvement in health was seen as instrumental in the achievement of some further purpose, such as raising productivity or contributing to social welfare. A number of the plans laid down explicit targets for health service coverage of the population; in a fifth of plans there were quantified targets for changes in health status indicators and about as frequently (though generally not involving the same countries) there were quantified targets for reductions in fertility or the population growth rate. For example, the Sierra Leone National Development Plan 1974/75–1978/79 postulated changes in the crude death rate, infant mortality rate, and life expectancy, but not fertility; the Third Malaysia Plan had no mortality targets, but announced a specific fertility target, the reduction of the crude birth rate from 31 to 28 per thousand over the plan period (1976–1980).

In reviewing the details of the specific policy measures adopted in the plans, an element of caution is necessary. The lack of explicit mention of a particular service does not necessarily mean that such a service is not provided or that concern for it does not exist. Some plans may include incomplete abstraction or inconsistent passages from the original plan documents; generic terms such as 'logistic support' or 'preventive services' are used in some plans where others itemize the components of these concepts; and some of the plan documents are merely summaries of the full plan translated into English (e.g. Korea, Turkey) which inevitably omit some of the details of the originals.

None the less, it is still highly relevant to study the content of the plans and to attempt to capture their main emphases. Virtually all the plans listed measures to strengthen the system of basic health services as a high priority, indeed in more than a third of the plans this appeared as the first priority. On the other hand, relatively few plans referred to the concept of primary care provided through village health workers (perhaps partly because this is a relatively recent policy emphasis); specific mention was found only in the plans of India, Indonesia, Pakistan, Sudan, and Thailand. Family planning was a major concern in more than half the plans and was the first priority of the Iran and Philippines plans. Family planning services are often envisaged as an integrated component of maternal and child health services (MCH), though in a number of countries without a strong commitment to family planning, MCH alone received a high priority. Overall, there were eight mentions of MCH in conjunction with family planning and four mentions of MCH alone as a priority programme.

Nutrition was identified as a priority programme in thirteen countries, water supply and sanitation in sixteen and health education in eleven. The persistence of traditional concerns such as communicable disease control (most frequently malaria) and development of hospital services was reflected in the high proportion of plans which mentioned these as priorities: 16 and 27 respectively. In nearly a third of the plans, hospital developments appeared as the first priority. However, the changing pattern of morbidity in developing countries was reflected in the interest shown in mental, dental, occupational health, and rehabilitation services not only in the richer and more sophisticated, but also in some of the poorest, developing countries.

Common to many of the plans was a high level of recognition of the need for support services. Virtually all the plans gave training and manpower development as a priority area, and in two (Botswana, Guyana) it was the first priority. There were only four plans which specifically distinguished medical education as a priority, but this count clearly understates the degree of commitment and/or concern, since in most of these countries medical education is the formal responsibility of the Ministry of Education, through whom the necessary budgetary allocations are made. Research as an input to the planning of services was mentioned in only three plans, though the need to develop statistical services was identified in thirteen and enhancement of planning capacity in three.

The need for restructuring or better management of services was identified in no less than 17 plans.

This account of current health sectoral planning and development planning supports the claim that the preoccupations of health planners are largely distinct from those of national economic planners. There are certain points of tangency: both are interested in family planning, though from different standpoints. The macro-planners attach greater weight to the impact of high fertility on variables such as the volume of savings and the pattern of investment, the dependency burden and the labour market, whereas health planners tend to justify the same allocations to family planning programmes by reference to the benefits of lower infant and maternal mortality and morbidity. The concern of macro-planners with an equitable distribution of income is paralleled by the concern of health planners to make health services more accessible to the population by the reduction of geographical and institutional barriers to their use.

These instances apart, however, it would appear the health planners operate in a context encapsulated from the macro-economic concerns with the growth of income, savings, and investment, with the changing sectoral composition of output and the strain on the balance of payments. The main point of contact is provided by the budgetary allocations for public sector health services, whose fluctuations transmit the backwash from the vagaries of the national economy. The function which health planners seek to optimize is clearly sector-specific. The objective of maximizing the output of 'health', subject to resource and other constraints, is common to all the sectoral plans. The output of 'health' is variously interpreted as the production of health services (which might more appropriately be regarded as a form of intermediate output) or the enhancement of health status, but it seems clear that this difference arises only from the close identification of health service production with better health. The successful implementation of health plans is measurable in terms of mortality and morbidity indicators; it is neither possible (nor from the standpoint of health planners does it seem necessary, or even desirable) to transpose improvements in mortality and morbidity into other measures of value.

The methodology of health planning

There are two significant differences between planning for the health sector and planning other sectors of the economy. In other sectors, the first stage of the planning process is to estimate demand, which is assumed to be exogenously determined, and the second stage is to devise a production plan to meet the demand. In the health sector, the first stage is to determine what the programmed demand of the sector ought to be—the determination of demand is endogenous to the planned process. The fundamental reason why health planners find it necessary to look behind the demand curve is that they generally perceive their function as the optimization of the health status of the population, and not of the output of the health services industry. In this perspective, a distinction may be made between planning health services and planning for health, or comprehensive health planning, the latter recognizing the multiple influences additional to health services which impinge on health status. Even within this perspective, it may be perfectly rational for health planners to concentrate on the provision of medical services if they judge such interventions to be more productive than equivalent resource outlays directed at alternative programmes.

Pragmatic planning

Very little health planning in developing countries has hitherto been accomplished with the assistance of formal, systematic methodologies. The great bulk of planning activity has been in the tradition of pragmatic or empirical planning. Within this tradition, three sub-types may be distinguished:

(1) project planning;
(2) integrated health services planning; and
(3) comprehensive sectoral planning.

To some extent, these sub-types represent both a progression of plan sophistication and an evolutionary path that some countries have followed through successive planning efforts.

Many early plans and a few current ones consist of little more than a list of proposals for capital expenditure on discrete projects in the government health service. (In this respect, the health sector plan usually reflects a national development plan which is merely a public sector investment plan.) It is characteristic of plans of this type that they lack coherence. Frequently there is no detailed statement of objectives and, if there is, the actual selection of projects typically does not reflect the declared priorities. There are few, if any, linkages between projects; each project is justified individually, rather than in terms of its contribution to an overall conception. There is a general lack of clear criteria for project selection; often the only justification offered is an assertion of necessity (often based on the consensus judgement of informed professionals, conscious of the deficiencies of existing services), but with no attempt to quantify the expected benefit. If any such quantification is attempted, it is generally expressed in terms of an expansion of capacity or supply of services, reflecting intermediate, rather than final, output. Such planning employs neither epidemiological information nor epidemiological calculation. Typically, it concerns itself exclusively with government health services, ignoring both health services provided under other auspices (such as the private sector and voluntary agencies) and health-promoting programmes in related sectors. Even within the area of government health services, the plans lack logistical consistency; for example, it is routine for the construction of health service premises to run ahead of the supply of trained staff to man them and the recurrent finance to keep them stocked with drugs and consumable supplies. This style of planning, a form of that mode of planning known as 'disjointed incrementalism', has been both criticized and commended. Its most evident virtue is flexibility, since almost any collection of activities can be designated as a project. The most obvious weakness of project-by-project planning, from the standpoint of optimal resource allocation in the health sector, is the absence of a criterion by which to evaluate and rank individual projects. It is widely understood that the noncommensurability of some of the project costs and benefits precludes the use of rate-of-return tests which can be applied to other public services, such as roads; it is less frequently understood that even a more limited ranking—by tests of cost effectiveness—is only feasible among alternatives producing very similar outputs. A formal test of cost-effectiveness is therefore unhelpful in choosing the preferred project if the candidates are a disease eradication project, a health centre construction programme and a manpower training programme, because each yields substantially different forms of output.

Nevertheless, the lack of common units of output is not a complete bar to project selection. Decision-makers do find it possible to rank alternatives; in so doing, they are presumably making a rough judgement of cost-effectiveness, that the preferred alternative makes a greater contribution to the improvement of the health of the nation than other potential uses of the same resources. However vaguely and inconsistently, decision-makers do hold a mental picture of a social welfare function, and do estimate crudely the productivity of alternative uses of resources. The cause for concern is that, given the paucity of quantified analysis, the area for discretionary judgement is so large that the uninformed opinions of political and professional leaders may effectively dominate the resource allocation process.

At first sight it might appear that the weaknesses of project (or incremental) planning are obviated by forms of integrated health services planning. This approach to planning does indeed display a number of marked advantages over project planning: typically, it envisages the development of a coherent structure of services, taking cognisance of the contribution of non-government providers as well as central and local government; generally there is a greater emphasis on the logistical consistency of the sectoral plan, so that increments in plant capacity are matched by increments in the supply of trained staff and consumable supplies. The justification for individual projects is then framed in terms of their contribution towards the overall structure of services. This does not mean that there is no need to choose between alternative uses of resources, but merely that the crucial allocation decisions are taken in the course of the design of the ultimate structure of services. Hence, there is still a need to choose, for example, between institutional and community-based services, between different combinations of professional, auxiliary, and volunteer workers, between personal and environmental services.

One important difference is that in integrated health services planning the decisions are taken simultaneously rather than serially; another is that the formulation of plans is usually preceded by a situation analysis which takes into account not only the epidemiological picture but also the total availability of resources over a period of time. Two clear advantages stem from this simultaneous consideration of alternatives; first, by widening the range of potential alternatives to each proposal, the chances are diminished of a still better alternative being overlooked, so the ranking of decisions should be more consistent. Secondly, it is much easier to take account of the complementarity which exists between projects.

While optimum resource allocation requires in principle that each discrete use of resources should be compared with all potential alternatives, in practice this procedure is too cumbersome and a simplifying device is used in integrated planning. Broad strategic decisions are made first, mostly relating to physical facilities and the manpower categories to be employed by the health service, and these decisions set the framework for more detailed planning on the precise content of those services. By contrast, in project planning, broad strategy (if it can be discerned at all) represents the accumulation of a series of individual unrelated decisions. An example which may suggest how, under identical material circumstances, these different planning procedures might result in different plans, is provided by the proposal to introduce a series of immunization programmes: in the project-by-project approach, the high costs of setting up the infrastructure to achieve high coverage of the population would be noted and compared with the benefits of each programme serially; in the integrated planning approach, the substantial element of joint costs would be noted and developing the capacity to deliver a complete immunization schedule could be seen as an attractive strategic choice.

The chief connection between macroeconomic planning and health planning in either of these two approaches is the budgetary limit imposed by government on capital and recurrent spending. Indeed, in one planning exercise, the *only* guidance furnished to those drafting the health sector plan by the central planning agency was a set of expenditure ceilings. As is implied by the term empirical or pragmatic planning, this style readily accommodates policy objectives derived from wider national considerations, such as giving priority to industries and localities earning foreign exchange, or to developing services in backward areas to change regional income distribution.

The additional element in comprehensive sectoral planning, compared with integrated health services planning, is an appreciation of the multiple determinants of health status and a corresponding recognition of the possibility of achieving favourable interventions through action in many sectors in addition to action affecting health services. However, the range of data required is enormously extended, embracing not only the epidemiological and operational statistics needed for health services planning, but also a wide range of economic, social, and technological observations and forecasts. Trends in nutrition, family structure, settlement patterns, and employment are scanned and their association with epidemiological measures assessed with a view to identifying health policies designed to ameliorate the health outcomes.

The scope of the policy interventions is equally wide, from direct provision of services in health-related sectors such as water supply, through food subsidies and taxes on alcohol and tobacco, to legal regulation of food hygiene, building standards, and industrial safety, in addition to the development of conventional health services. Much of this planning activity is interdisciplinary and intersectoral, effected by health ministry representation on interdepartmental committees and by the provision of advice to other agencies, rather than by the production of blueprints for action by the health service hierarchy. Because the instruments of policy are not always under the direct control of government health services, planners need to become advocates for the health interest in every relevant sphere of social policy (as has been argued for nutrition, see, for instance, Chapter 9).

Formal planning methodologies

Pragmatic planning represents those styles of planning which have evolved over time in response to practical experience. In addition, a limited number of formal health planning methodologies have been developed. A common feature of such methodologies is often that, in choosing preferred interventions among a range of possible candidates, it is suggested that a crude or implicit test of cost-effectiveness be used by professional and political decision-makers. However, it is not at first sight always apparent how the resource constraint is imported into the decision process. For instance, in the official accounts of health planning in the USSR (Popov 1971; Bogatyrev and Rojtman 1972) emphasis is given to the technical nature of the planning process, that is health services are planned to respond to morbidity, using techniques which have been assessed through operational research. On close examination of the sequence of planning operations, it becomes evident that the necessary adjustment to resource availability is effected by determining the design standards (*normativ* in Russian) and creating an 'equilibrium' between the various subdivisions of the public health plan and also between the public health plan and the national economic plan. It appears that in the process of setting the design standards for each service, due account is taken of the resource cost implications and, furthermore, in giving some services relatively generous standards, resources are allocated to those uses which are considered to be most efficient in the sense of most cost-effective.

The PAHO–CENDES method (Ahumada 1965; Hilleboe, Barkhuus, and Thomas 1972) quite explicitly uses a test of cost-effectiveness as the basis for resource allocation in the health sector. This methodology, which in a number of important respects was a forerunner of the World Health Organization's current model of country health programming, relies on an extensive epidemiological data input and concentrates its concern upon the productivity of various resource inputs. It overtly recognizes that there are finite resources available to the health sector and that there is, therefore, a need to compare alternative potential uses for these limited resources. It proposes that:

The general rule for allocating resources is that they should be allocated in such a way as to obtain a maximum product per resource unit used and the proof that this standard is being attained is in the impossibility of further increasing production by transferring a resource from one use to another . . . We propose in this document to identify the use with the disease, or more generally speaking, with a given hazard to health. The problem then consists in how to allocate the resources available from year to year to control the various diseases . . . In principle, all diseases are arranged according to the cost of preventing a death and the resources available are allocated to combat the disease that appears in first position until it is reduced to a level that the most efficient technique permits. Any resources left over are then allocated to the disease in second place, and so on down the line (Ahumada 1965).

Not surprisingly, perhaps, the PAHO—CENDES method has been found to be extremely difficult to apply in practice. Notwithstanding its apparently rational approach, one obvious difficulty is that the resource allocation criterion adopted refers to only one form of output (reduction of mortality) whereas most health programmes produce multiple impacts. A second issue is that, except for a few disease-specific programmes, it is difficult to allocate resources to single diseases, rather than to a service or facility that may then be deployed against many disease problems.

The latest national health planning methodology to emerge under WHO auspices, Country Health Programming, can be viewed as an attempt to accommodate these and other deficiencies of the prototype (WHO 1979a). It gets over the problem of noncommensurable outputs by defining the output of health programmes in terms of 'problem reduction', and by allowing problems to be defined in terms other than exclusively diagnostic categories. It is also realistic in its assumptions of the political and administrative context within which health sector resource allocations are made. However, in its original form it was less than clear on the decision criteria to be used in selecting priority health programmes. The sequence of steps implied that detailed costing of programmes would only be undertaken after the programmes had been chosen and formulated in some detail, which is difficult to reconcile with the use of a cost-effectiveness criterion in selecting the priorities. In the light of a review of national experiences in applying country health programming (WHO 1979b) three broad stages up to the point of programme adoption are now envisaged, in which the resource requirements are progressively refined. The first stage is formulation of general health policies, strategies, and plans of action, and entails obtaining indicative (or order of magnitude) commitments on funding, subject to later acceptance of detailed programmes. The second stage is broad programming, in which long-term strategic plans with time-phased objectives and targets are developed, and the medium-term budgetary implications of strategies for system change and service delivery are calculated. The third stage is detailed programme formulation, which specifies the tactics, the detailed technologies to be used and the types of resources required.

The matching of technical actions and resource specifications with timed targets of accomplishment permits the formulation of annual budgets so as to convert indicator allocations into firm approvals of programme funding (WHO, 1979*b*).

There can be little doubt that, presented in this way, Country Health Programming represents a substantial gain in the feasibility of the planning process which now corresponds broadly to the historic practice of empirical comprehensive planning.

Although the methodologies of health sectoral planning have been developed largely in isolation from the mainstream of national development planning, they do echo some common concerns. The last decade and a half has seen the evolution of integrated systems of project appraisal, which seek to relate the objectives of national development planning to the selection of individual projects (OECD 1968; UNIDO 1972; Little and Mirrlees 1974; Squire and Van der Tak 1975). These systems of project appraisal were designed for application to the directly productive sectors of the economy, and cannot usefully be applied to investment in social infrastructure. Nevertheless, the same themes which have inspired the development of health planning methodologies—the emphasis on efficiency and equity in resource allocation, the consistent application of selection criteria, the circumspect regard for adverse and unintended consequential effects of policies—are clearly the inspiration of the project appraisal methodologies. However, it must be doubted whether the future will see any greater convergence. While the benefits of health expenditures remain resistant to expression in common units of welfare, goals for the health sector will need to be set in sector-specific terms, and the process of optimizing goal achievement is likely to retain its enclave character.

Conclusion

The gulf between national development planning and health sectoral planning has been amply demonstrated. The adverse consequences of the divide are much more difficult to demonstrate. There is no discernible connection between the degree of sophistication of macroeconomic planning and the scale of resources devoted to the health sector or the efficiency of their use. There is a presumption that greater sophistication in sectoral planning is associated both with relatively larger allocations of resources to health and their more effective deployment. At present, the state of the art of development planning and development models hardly permits a judgement on the overall gain in welfare that may result from a reallocation of resources in favour of the health sector. One can be more confident that there is considerable scope for welfare gains from the more efficient use of any given level of resources and, given widespread evidence of existing misallocation in developing countries (even within the objectives publicly subscribed by political decision-makers), it is probable that the best return on the investment in health planning endeavour over the next few years will be found in intrasectoral initiatives, to refine and improve health planning methodologies and, in particular, to make them more sensitive to cost, efficiency, and effectiveness considerations.

REFERENCES

Ahumada, J. (1965). Health planning: problems of concept and method. *Scientific Publication No. 111.* Pan American Health Organization, Washington DC.

Bogatyrev, I. D. and Rojtman, M. P. (1972). Public health planning in the USSR. In Approaches to national health planning (ed. H. E. Hilleboe *et al.*). *Publ. Hlth Pap. WHO* **46.**

Clark, P. G. (1965). *Development planning in East Africa.* East African Publishing House, Nairobi.

Feldstein, M. S. (1970). Health sector planning in developing countries. *Economica* **37,** 139–63.

Frederiksen, H. (1969). Feedbacks in economic and demographic transition. *Science, NY* **166,** 837–47.

Grosse, R. N. (1980). Interrelation between health and population: observations derived from field experiences. *Social Sci. Med.* **14C,** 99–120.

Hilleboe, H. E., Barkhuus, A., and Thomas, W. C. (1972). Approaches to national health planning. *Publ. Hlth Pap. WHO,* **46.**

Little, I. M. D. and Mirrlees, J. A. (1974). *Project appraisal and planning for developing countries.* Heinemann Educational Books, London.

OECD (Organization for Economic Co-operation and Development) (1968). *Manual of industrial project analysis in developing countries* Vol. II, Social cost–benefit analysis. Organization for Economic Co-operation and Development, Paris.

Popov, G. A. (1971). Principles of health planning in the USSR. *Publ. Hlth Pap. WHO* **43.**

Squire, L. and Van der Tak, H. G. (1975). *Economic analysis of projects.* Johns Hopkins University Press, Baltimore.

Taylor, C. E. and Hall, M. F. (1967). Health, population and economic development. *Science, NY* **157,** 651–7.

Tinbergen, J. (1967). *Development planning.* World University Library, London.

Todaro, M. P. (1971). *Development planning.* Oxford University Press, Nairobi.

UNIDO (United Nations Industrial Development Organization) (1972). *Guidelines for project evaluation.* United Nations Industrial Development Organization, New York.

WHO (World Health Organization) (1973). Interrelationships between health programmes and socio-economic development. *Publ. Hlth Pap. WHO* **49.**

— (1979*a*). *Working guidelines for country health programming.* CHP/IRS/79.5. World Health Organization, Geneva.

— (1979*b*). *Applying country health programming.* **MPP/CHP** 79.2. World Health Organization, Geneva.

11

The economics of health in developing countries: a critical review

Kenneth Lee and Anne Mills

Introduction

This final chapter does not address itself to high theory or to complex methodologies; nor does it offer any detailed illumination of key economic concepts. In other chapters, authors have explored their own particular areas of interest, and this chapter therefore attempts to draw together these various strands, to clarify the role of economists and economics in the formulation of health policies and in influencing an evaluation of health strategies appropriate to the requirements of developing countries. Differences between developing countries are certainly not unimportant, but the distinction between countries in Europe, North America, and Australasia and those in Asia, Africa, and South America is clear. It is to their similarities and common problems that this book has been addressed.

This chapter argues that in developing countries the financial climate is encouraging governments and health workers to exhibit a close interest in the economics of health and health care. There is already evidence of a growing willingness to employ or request economists to analyse systematically the allocation of resources to and within the health sector. At the same time, there has been considerable discussion amongst health economists about the nature and value of the contribution which they and their sub-discipline (of health economics) can make to an understanding of health problems and the manner of their resolution.

This chapter is in five main parts. First, a glossary of economic concepts is presented to help the reader and to demonstrate that economics does possess certain ideas, distinct from other disciplines, which can be of considerable value to health planners and managers alike. It is hoped that this list is a useful one, for it is difficult for economists to remove all professional terms from their writings. Second, many of the key questions that should be of close interest to policy-makers, and the relevant economic concepts and techniques which could be applied to them, are set out in tabular form. These tables are amplified in the third section, which focuses on the conceptual and methodological problems likely to be faced by those wishing to apply economic reasoning to the health sector.

The chapter then moves on from analysis to consider implementation, and investigates the political and institutional constraints and barriers to the acceptance of economic analysis in the health sector. In the past, some have considered it improper to apply the philosophy of economics and economic techniques to health, for instance in the belief that services should be made available to those for whom they may be beneficial, as a matter of right without regard to economics. Today, however much politicians and health professions may regret it, economics is of increasing importance in the management of health expenditure. Slogans aimed at keeping economics out of health, or health out of economics, are misplaced when governments involve themselves directly or indirectly in the health sector. Finally, therefore, this chapter aims to clarify what role the economist can play in the health sector of developing countries; to document the ways in which economics can be applied to a broad spectrum of health care issues at both the macro and micro levels; and to respond to the key question, namely how best can economists and economics help policy-makers and others improve the future welfare of populations?

The relevant corpus of economics

The potential contribution of economic principles to an understanding of the health sector of developing countries is well illustrated by the definition of economics provided in Chapter 1: the study of how people and society end up choosing, with or without the use of money, to employ scarce productive resources . . . to produce various commodities and distribute them for consumption, now or in the future, among various people and groups in society. This definition suggests that economics and economists should be interested in issues of policy choice in health, in analysing alternative methods of providing a desired service or outcome, in time scale, and in rationing and distribution.

Certain key economic concepts and techniques are basic to the economist's approach to these issues, and a glossary appears below that policy-makers, health planners, and health workers might find useful in relating economics to their own areas of responsibility. The list is not exhaustive, but gives a good indication of many of the ideas with which contributors to this volume have been concerned in analysing the health sector. Although the terms themselves may be unfamiliar, the narrative has been drafted for the non-economist; no attempt is made to explain the underlying economic theories and models.

Scarcity

Some might claim that health care is so essential to life that it must be provided regardless of cost; and that doctors and other health workers must act in the best interests of their patients and communities and not be influenced by economic or financial considerations. The counter-argument is that 'scarcity' exists in all walks of life, that no-one can buy everything they would like to, and that there is no such thing as free food, water, or medical care. It follows that the economist's notion of scarcity is of particular importance, for the health needs of the developing countries are for all practical purposes infinite, while their resources are so clearly limited.

Opportunity cost

This simple but important concept affirms that the real cost to a society of providing a health service is its 'opportunity cost', since the manpower and resources employed are made unavailable for other purposes. Hence, given scarcity of resources, the economist seeks to find out not only what something costs in money terms, but also what sacrifices it implies in terms of doing without other things. If from the available budget it is possible to provide either service A or service B but not both, then the cost of acquiring A is that B is sacrificed. This is important information when combined with judgements about the relative benefits of A and B.

The scarcer the resources the higher will be the opportunity costs. Thus one possible approach for the health planner or policy-maker is to ask: 'what is the least valuable thing we are doing?' and 'what is the most valuable thing we are not doing?', and seek to shift the resources if the latter is greater than the former. This same approach can be adopted by the doctor, the pharmacist, or the community health volunteer, to ask 'what difference will it make if I decide to provide (or to continue to provide) this service, and what are the alternatives?' By asking what difference it will make, one is asking the health worker to think about the extent to which the service is, or will be, beneficial to patients; and by asking about alternatives, one is asking the health worker to consider always that scarce resources can be used for other purposes and for other patients.

Costs

It follows that economists will wish to identify all the resource implications of health sector activities, and not solely the money 'costs'. In consequence, the economist is interested not only in what a health activity will cost (say) the government sector, but also what hidden or unquantifiable costs are imposed on the patient, the patient's family and relatives, the local community and on other agencies. Attempts to identify and value the costs of health services should at the very least recognize that there are costs incurred by both providers and consumers, in terms of the resources they expend in delivering or consuming health care.

Production function

The term 'production function' is an expression of the relationship between inputs and outputs, and represents a tool for analysing how different resources (inputs), such as doctors, health workers, and community volunteers, can be combined to produce services (outputs) of various kinds. In other words, each production function has its own specific inputs and outputs.

Different ways exist to provide a good or service and to treat a patient. A policy-relevant question is what are the technical and financial options for substitution? The degree of substitutability between different types of resources (for instance recurrent and capital), or between different types of health worker (for instance doctor, health worker, volunteer) is important to determine, since it provides information the policy-maker needs to know in order to minimize the costs of providing effective health care. The concept of the production function is equally applicable to activities not directly providing patient care, such as the construction of sanitation facilities, health centres, dispensaries, or hospitals, which may be produced by different methods, using different materials, at different levels of cost. Hence, the production function describes what it is possible to achieve from different resource combinations: it is, in essence, a shopping list from which policy-makers, planners, and managers can choose their 'best buys'.

Demand

The economist's concept of demand is rooted in the notion of what a person is *able* and *willing* to pay. Demand is seen to reflect both the strength of the person's desire to receive the service, that is the value placed on it, and the amount that will have to be sacrificed in order to do so. However, the immediate relevance of this concept of 'demand' may be far from clear in those countries whose basic health services are provided free or at subsidized prices. A community's demand for primary health care or a potable water supply does none the less only exist in terms of what that community is prepared to sacrifice in money, time, inconvenience, and incidental costs incurred. In the economics literature, 'demand' is sometimes termed 'expressed' need in order to separate it conceptually from 'self-perceived' need or from 'professionally defined' need. Of course, the utilization of health services does not depend solely upon demand; rather, it is the result of the interaction of demand and supply, of consumers and providers, though they do not necessarily interact on equal terms.

Elasticity

The economist's notion of 'elasticity' is one which can be applied to both the demand and the supply of health services and health-promoting activities. On the *demand* side, the concept describes the degree of responsiveness of a person's demand for, say, medical treatment to a change in his income (income elasticity) or to a change in the charge he has to pay (price elasticity). For example, by how much are people likely to reduce their use of a particular drug if its cost to them increases? The degree to which demand is elastic (that is, sensitive to price changes) will depend upon the availability of substitutes, since if one form of health care (such as a drug) has close substitutes, a rise in its price (relative to the prices of substitutes) to consumers could reduce the level of its demand considerably. On the *supply* side, the concept is used to reflect the ease or difficulty with which it is possible to change the volume of health services provided, or the ease with which medical and nursing services, drugs, etc., can be substituted for each other. The elasticity of supply also depends upon substitutes, so that if various forms of health worker are close substitutes for each other in the tasks they can perform, a reduction in the level of remuneration for one is likely to reduce the demand for similar forms of health worker by making them relatively more expensive.

The margin

The economist recognizes that most policy changes in the health sector, and most managerial decisions, will take place at the 'margin'; that is to say, decisions will rarely be concerned with totally eliminating one health activity and starting up a completely new one, but rather with doing less of one, and a little more of another. Hence most decisions will be at the margin, and should follow a consideration of what the cost and benefits will be of expanding or contracting existing services.

Shadow pricing

The intention of 'shadow pricing' is to estimate a price which is as close an approximation as possible of the real value of the resources used in the health sector; that is which reflects their true scarcity. Shadow pricing can be used to determine a price for costs and benefits in circumstances either where no prices exist, or where the prices that do exist are considered to be an imperfect indicator of the value of the costs incurred or benefits received. In developing countries, the general effect of applying shadow pricing to the costing of health activities is to emphasize the relative merits of those options that use the greatest proportions of low-skilled labour (such as auxiliary workers whose actual wage may overstate their opportunity cost) and home produced materials (such as domestically produced drugs and vaccines which save on expensive foreign exchange). In addition, if inequalities in health are a primary concern and are considered to be highly correlated with poverty, then health care benefits to some groups (for instance the poor) might be given a greater value (or weight) in any policy analysis. Alternatively, costs could be given less weight, with the objective of reducing the implied cost of health programmes targeted at the lowest income groups and thus favouring their selection.

Externalities

The term 'externality' is used by economists to describe third-party, community, or spill-over effects of activities which occur either through the operation of the market but are not taken into account in production decisions or prices charged for goods or services, or which result from the activities of public bodies. It can be appropriate for governments to curtail or reduce activities that generate 'external' costs (such as the costs to society of environmental pollution) through direct controls and taxes, and to promote those activities that generate 'external' benefits, that is which benefit more people than the immediate recipients (such as immunization programmes) by direct subsidies and/or public provision.

Equity

In the health sector, as in most walks of life, there is a potential conflict between quantity and quality, and between primary health care for all and high technology medicine for the few. High technology services, if they are also high cost services, inevitably mean few beneficiaries and inadequate coverage for the populations of the developing world. When countries aim to improve the health of their population, a key question for them is the meaning of 'equity': does it mean equal access to health facilities, equal use of services, or equal health status? Should health planning be concerned with efficiency, in terms of using resources to greatest effect, or with fair shares for all? Likewise, does fairness when applied to the health sector mean distributing services in relation to need regardless of income, or does it mean that people should pay for health care in direct proportion to their income and wealth?

Cost-effectiveness analysis

One of the newer tools of health policy analysis is 'cost-effectiveness analysis', which aims to ascertain one of two things: either the health programme capable of achieving specified objectives at the lowest possible cost (for instance the lowest cost per life saved); or the programme which will maximize the benefit to be gained from a given health budget (for instance the greatest number of lives saved). In either case one of the parameters is fixed, and the aim is simply to maximize the benefit or to minimize the cost. The price to be paid for this simplicity is that the analysis cannot show whether the objectives were worth achieving in the first place, in comparison with other possible objectives.

Cost-benefit analysis

Since resources in developing countries will always be limited, criteria are required to help make a considered choice of whether to provide some services and refrain from undertaking other services. Some health services and health-related activities are more effective in promoting health than others. Economists stress that an appropriate criterion is that resources should be spent on those activities which bring the greatest benefit in relation to their costs.

'Cost-benefit analysis' has developed, therefore, as a method of approach for applying this criterion, to examine the disadvantages and advantages of alternative policy options, and the efficacy and cost of individual tests and treatments. The cost-benefit method attempts to value all relevant costs and outcomes over periods of time in order to help decide whether or not, when costs and benefits are identified, measured, and valued, a particular strategy is worth adopting. The basic idea of cost-benefit analysis is a very simple one: it sets out to discover the extent to which the benefits of a particular strategy outweigh its real (that is its opportunity) costs.

The scope of health economics

All the contributors to this book have demonstrated why health care and health cannot be exempted from the attention of economics and health economists. The basic claim of economics, as a social science, is that it can be of considerable help in determining, at all levels of policy-making, the optimal allocation of scarce resources among various alternatives. For example, in the context of many developing countries, is it more appropriate to commit funds to building a hospital or to setting up a number of health centres? Will local communities benefit more if the low-cost training of health workers and community volunteers is expanded rather than the high-cost training of doctors and professions supplementary to medicine? What are the costs and benefits of a vertical programme of immunization in comparison to the costs and benefits of a horizontal programme providing primary health care? Are efforts best directed to improving sanitation and providing safe drinking water or to bettering nutrition through improved agricultural production and distribution methods?

Table 11.1 places these kinds of questions within a uniform framework and explores the common ground between economics and health policy. The first column of the table identifies a number of 'health policy issues' that are of pressing concern to developing countries (items *I-X* inclusive). The economist, in examining such issues, will reflect on a set of further questions before the policy issues themselves can be tackled. These appear in the second column under the heading 'some prior questions'. The final column of Table 11.1, headed 'relevant corpus of economics', offers pointers to those parts of economic theory and those concepts and techniques which can be used to analyse the various planning and management issues identified. The purpose of presenting this table is to show that the issues are amenable to economic analysis, and to demonstrate that economics can and does bear upon a wide spectrum of health care issues that are central to the concerns of developing countries. Further, by tabulating the material in this way, it is hoped to encourage policy-makers, planners, and managers to identify those policy issues where they feel health economics and economists might be of greatest assistance to them.

State of the art

Table 11.1 is not intended to convey the impression that all the health policy issues identified (*I-X* inclusive) are currently the subject of sustained effort by economists, and that solutions to these issues are already to hand. This is not the case. Chapter 1 has already indicated that the economics of health and health care, as a sub-discipline of economics, is relatively new, dating largely from the early 1960s. Significant strides have been made since then in terms of both theoretical developments and empirical work, but much remains unexplored. What follows here is not so much an assessment of the achievements of the sub-discipline (the reader can judge those for himself or herself), but rather a reflection on the efforts still needed and the conceptual and technical

TABLE 11.1. *The relevance of economics to the health sector*

Some health policy issues	Some prior questions	Relevant corpus of economics
I. Health and economic development (health and health care as determinant and consequence of socioeconomic development)	1. What constitutes health and health improvement? 2. What are the determinants of health improvement? 3. How does health (and health services) affect production and the economy?	Identification and measurement issues of health and illness/disease; basic needs measures. Macroeconomic models of economic development; determinants of growth. Human capital theory: investment and consumption elements of health expenditure; household production functions for health; ill-health and the productivity of labour
II. Organization and delivery systems (structure of health care and health-related activities)	1. What are the economic characteristics of health care and health-related activities? 2. What is the relevance of these characteristics for the pursuit of health through market and non-market mechanisms? 3. How do different health care systems handle their organization and distribution decisions?	Welfare theory and market failure: rationality, consumer sovereignty, income and wealth issues, indivisibilities, externalities, public goods and merit goods
III. Finance of the health sector (income aspects of health care and health-related activities)	1. What are the sources of health care financing? 2. What type and quantity of resources are being utilized to finance the health sector? 3. What do alternative financing methods achieve both in terms of yield and of incidence (burden)?	Social accounting systems and public finance: revenue generation and tax incidence; self-financing, insurance and pre-payment mechanisms; ability and willingness-to-pay concepts

TABLE 11.1 (*cont.*)

Some health policy issues	Some prior questions	Relevant corpus of economics
IV. Demand analysis (the demand and need for health and health services)	1. What determines the demand (or absence of demand) for specific health services, and for traditional healers, herbalists, and practitioners? 2. What factors determine the provider response to an individual's demands for health care, including factors such as the availability of referral facilities? 3. How do health payment systems (e.g. charges, pre-payment methods) affect the demand for and utilization of health services?	Theories of household, individual and supplier-induced behaviour: generation and interpretation of demand schedules; determinants of demand, price, income, and cross-elasticities; time costs
V. Supply analysis (physical resources and costs)	1. What determines the cost behaviour of organizations and health agencies? 2. How and why will costs vary with changes in the scale, location, or type of medical and health services (and facilities) provided? 3. What mix of resources will produce specific services?	Production functions and substitutability between inputs. Estimation of short- and long-run cost curves, average and marginal costs, private and social costs. Determinants of hospital and health centre cost variations (case-mix, quality factors); economies of scale
VI. Health manpower (human resources: their availability, motivation and remuneration)	1. What determines the supply and distribution of each type of human resource? 2. How do forms of remuneration and other determinants of behaviour affect manpower recruitment, absenteeism, retention, and geographical distribution? 3. What are the productivities of various types of health worker in relation to their training costs and rates of pay?	Labour markets and the demand for and supply of health workers. Marginal productivity theory. Factors influencing supply elasticities: impact of income levels and financial incentives, leisure preferences; private practice; the brain drain

VII. Financial management
(cost containment and cost efficiency)

1. How is the budget divided, who controls the budget, and how is that control exercised?
2. Can economies be effected in the procurement and distribution of resources?
3. What is an 'appropriate' technology?

Budgeting systems and accountability (cost centres, cost units); inventory management

Determinants of supplier behaviour (local, national, multi-national)

Shadow pricing and social opportunity costs

VIII. Organizational behaviour
(individual and corporate objectives and motives underpinning behaviour of health agencies)

1. Who makes the resource allocation decisions to and within the health sector, and what are their objectives?
2. What is the feasibility of reconciling the conflicting goals, values and interests of the various groups and individuals involved in the health sector?
3. What types of controls or incentives (monetary or otherwise) can be introduced to encourage efficient behaviour?

Managerial and behaviour theories of government, not-for-profit, profit and voluntary organizations

Notions of efficiency and the role of inducements (rewards and penalties)

IX. Project evaluation
(desirability and implications of reducing, expanding, or redeploying existing services, or introducing new activities)

1. Does the service do any good or have any discernible effect on health? For whom?
2. What are the relative efficiencies (merits and de-merits) of alternative health activities?
3. What are the distributional consequences of health activities (who incurs the cost, who receives the benefits?)

Managerial and behavioural theories of and cost-effective analyses. Notions of 'effectiveness' and the 'margin'; size and incidence of costs and benefits

X. Health policy, equity, and social justice
(providing the right services in the right places to the right people at the right time)

1. How best can resources be matched to the population's needs, mortality and morbidity patterns, demands and utilization?
2. What impact do different health care systems have upon eligibility, access, take-up, and benefits received by target groups in the population?
3. What are the barriers, if any, to the provision of an equitable (fair) health service?

Optimum welfare criteria and the concept of the social welfare function

Inequalities and inequities in health care: definition and measurement issues

Effect of socioeconomic variables and physical access on utilization patterns problems still to be faced and resolved. With that objective in mind, these ten policy issues provide a convenient way of structuring the discussion, in order to offer a personal assessment of the present state of the art of the economics of health in developing countries.

I. Health and economic development

The conceptual distinctions to be drawn between health, health services, and health-promoting activities are undoubtedly important ones, and it is also important to find an operational definition of the term 'health'. Though the task of determining suitable definitions lies largely outside the domain of economics, such definitions will none the less condition the analytical approaches economists adopt to determining the efficiency and effectiveness of the health sector. Once 'health' has been defined, the question 'what are the determinants of health?' can be asked. Health services are but one influence, and as Griffiths and Mills point out, there is now increased awareness of the many factors which influence health, particularly of activities which are not health services as such, but nevertheless are undertaken with the intention of improving health. However, it is proving extremely difficult to measure the specific contribution each activity makes to health; as Wheeler's chapter brings out very clearly, the relationship between a health service and health status is mediated by a host of environmental and behavioural factors, which are in turn influenced by almost every aspect of the social and natural systems.

In the context of a developing country which is trying to transform its economy and achieve rapid but equitable growth, the interrelationship between health and economic development is central to a consideration of health policy. As Cumper states, it is now widely agreed that there is an association between a country's place on the ladder of development and indicators of health such as life expectancy and infant mortality. However, Cumper stresses that many aspects of development cannot be classified as being favourable or unfavourable to health *per se*, but rather should be seen as having a wide range of possible effects, the outcome depending very much on the precise steps taken by governments. Hence, the policy implications of the relationship between economic development and health are often not clear. As Wheeler emphasizes, current models of development planning are not well adapted to incorporating the health sector in their projections. Governments in developing countries face a potential conflict between the use of additional public monies to expand the health sector and their use to increase the capital stock in the industrial sector. Wheeler and others in this volume have made plain that national planners may wish to propose restraint in the expansion of health services (which are assumed, in the absence of strong evidence to the contrary, to meet only current consumption needs), in order to permit greater investment to expand the economy's capacity to meet future consumption needs. It is therefore clear that the complexities of the interrelationships between health and economic development are neither well researched and documented nor well understood, and much work remains to be done.

II. Organization and delivery systems

What objectives are the organizational patterns and delivery systems of the health sector intended to achieve? In the absence of market forces which link together (however imperfectly and inequitably) production possibilities and consumer preferences, the economist wishes to be informed of the health objectives of society, and of the value that society places on health goals relative to other goals. However, the basic determinants, values, and assumptions underlying health planning, policy formulation, and decision-making are often not made explicit. As the chapters by Prescott and Warford, and Wheeler, remark, most health plans in developing countries formulate health objectives in terms of the expansion or improvement of health services rather than of health itself, perhaps not least because the health impact of particular inputs and interventions is rarely known with any certainty. Yet the objective of maximizing net benefit to society presupposes judgements about the relative weights to be given to different outcomes. For fear of political repercussions, policy-makers may be guarded or reluctant to confront these judgements explicitly.

Given the low level of articulation about what is to be maximized, there may well be imprecision and ambiguity about the appropriate role of the state versus the individual in matters of health policy and social welfare. Mills observes that the issues of why governments should intervene in the health care market, and whether on *a priori* grounds health care is most efficiently organized by the private or public sector, have long intrigued economists and produced a considerable theoretical debate. Clearly what matters are again the objectives a country seeks to achieve through its health sector and the means by which these can best be achieved. Governments, health workers, and various sections of the public will all have their own objectives and views. A major issue in the development process, as Ferster and Tilden emphasize, is therefore how to elicit the goodwill and sustained spirit and effort of everyone, including civil servants, communities, and the private health sector, to work towards national goals and objectives.

III. Finance of the health sector

No 'right' allocation of resources to the health sector can be established for the precise nature of the causal relationship between the size of a developing country's health expenditure and the state of its population's health is unclear. How much of any country's resources are devoted to government and private health services will be a matter for both political and individual decision. In the government sector, the magnitude of health expenditure results from the process of deciding the total of public expenditure, and then of allocating the total between competing programmes including health (Lee 1982a). The income of the private sector will depend on the demand of individual consumers and their interaction with providers.

Since resources are scarce and needs very great, there will always be a gap between the amount earmarked for a particular service and the amount that could be spent on it. Moreover, some sources of revenue are tied to financing certain services, or to providing care for certain groups of the population. For instance, as Lee argues, a reliance on local sources of fund raising and on local (as opposed to national) financing, can create disparities in the level and quality of care available and, other things being equal, in the quality of people's health, which reflect the relative wealth of different parts of a country. Another example of a means of financing and organizing health care which has equity implications is health insurance, selected for special attention by Mills. As she points out, some form of health insurance, involving contributions by individuals and/or employers, can prove extremely attractive to a health sector starved of funds and doubtful of getting resources from other quarters; but it can also finance high quality health care for a small proportion of the population.

In this regard, economic analyses of the sources of finance and of existing health expenditure patterns can provide important information for identifying efficient and equitable methods of mobilizing resources for the health sector. At present, as Prescott and Warford point out, health ministries are typically unaware of the detail of the allocation of public resources between different interventions and its relationship to stated health objectives, or of the unit costs of different interventions, or of the full potential of available sources of finance. By outlining a methodology for undertaking health sector financing and expenditure surveys in developing countries, Griffiths and Mills open up the possibility of further analytical work to show where the money comes from (sources of finance) in comparison with various classifications of how it is spent; to explore various alternatives, including health insurance, for financing health care; and to integrate this kind of work into the overall context of health planning and management.

IV. Demand analysis

How is the demand for health care determined? It is not easy, or indeed always relevant, to apply the traditional economic model of demand to the health sector. Major issues are to determine the relative importance to be attached to the concepts of 'need' and 'demand' in health policy determination, and to formulate theories of demand appropriate to the health sector. Undue emphasis on 'need' in the past has meant that evidence of what importance consumers place upon health and where they rank it alongside other consumer satisfactions is often lacking. More attempts could be made to tease out the processes by which people not only label themselves as 'in need', but also actively seek, and are prepared to pay for, health care (effective demand). As Lee concludes, the same combination of influences will not apply to all people, though financial, cultural, and organizational characteristics will all be important. Cumper raises the question of how far the relation between development and the consumption of health services can be accounted for in terms of income levels and the price of health care relative to other commodities on which consumers might spend their money. Certainly, the low level of incomes in the poorer developing countries is likely to mean that the health needs of a large part of the population are not translated into effective demand. For instance, Prescott and Warford raise doubts as to whether interventions such as primary health care, when directed at low income beneficiaries, will be effective under a system of direct user charges if potential consumers are deterred from seeking care by the level of prices charged. Likewise, as Westcott spells out, food and nutritional problems are as likely to stem from a lack of effective demand as from inadequate food production, or poor storage and distribution networks: a major underlying cause of hunger and malnutrition is that those who need food do not have the resources to buy it, not that it is unavailable. In summary, more detailed studies are required to explain how and why variations in demand for health care and health promoting goods and services are related to personal characteristics and to the characteristics of the various markets concerned.

V. Supply analysis

Health services and health-related activities range from simple low-cost services to complex and technologically sophisticated procedures. They are subject to various economic forces such as changes in input prices, changes in technical know-how, and changes in the pattern of demand. This complexity often frustrates attempts to define the health sector in terms of its production possibilities and its costs. For instance, in constructing a supply function of foodstuffs to the market, Westcott stresses the importance of also modelling aspects of the transport and distribution system which affect the market quantities available after they leave the farm; these include losses in storage, costs of transport, as well as the speculative behaviour of dealers who may withhold produce from the market if they believe that the price is about to rise.

There are limits to the amount any individual can afford to pay or any government is prepared to pay for health activities. It follows that in identifying production processes that are appropriate to local circumstances, an important economic factor is that of cost, since this will determine whether a given approach is or is not economically viable. There are usually more ways of carrying out a health programme than those options that health planners tend conventionally to consider, and alternative forms of supply will often require a trade-off to be made between cost and effectiveness. Earlier in this volume, Creese gave an example of such choices in immunization programmes: different vaccines, different vaccine schedules, different combinations of fixed centre or mobile outreach facilities, different degrees of integration with existing basic health services, and different types of immunization personnel were all examples of the alternative choices open to managers of immunization programmes.

VI. Health manpower

The emphasis in many recent national and international health policy statements has been upon the provision of preventive and promotive care through the primary health care approach. Yet in many developing countries the output of medical practitioners from university medical schools continues unabated; some doctors will expect to be employed by governments, others will want to migrate to the large cities, to practise privately, to undertake postgraduate training abroad, or to emigrate abroad. Whatever the merits of these options, little is known, as Ferster and Tilden state, about which precise set of manpower policy approaches might be most appropriate and efficient in addressing the health manpower needs faced by particular countries. However, it is clear that innovative strategies should be actively considered. These would focus on skills and technologies appropriate to local circumstances, and would be oriented towards the retention of health workers in their communities, located in the rural areas and poor urban settings where most of the population live, and practising from government health centres or on behalf of the local communities. Such a consideration involves identifying the opportunity costs of these various forms of health workers—both in terms of their cost (training, salary/activities foregone) and their effectiveness. As Lee argues in his chapter, the difference in the effectiveness of treatment for a wide range of ailments between a doctor and a community health worker is likely to be much less than the difference in the costs of their training and levels of remuneration. Much more analytical work is needed to identify how many types of manpower are, or could be, potential substitutes for each other, in both technical and financial terms.

VII. Financial management

Since limits will always be imposed on the amounts governments, health agencies and individuals feel able to allocate to the health sector, two features are of particular importance: the containment of costs and obtaining better value from existing resources. Central questions are likely to be who should control costs and be made accountable for expenditure, and how can efficiency be encouraged. With the objective of cost containment in mind and assuming that reliable cost data can be gathered, Prescott and Warford suggest that efficiency in service provision can be monitored by analysing trends in the unit costs of similar interventions at different points in time.

Such analysis provides a starting point for diagnosing inefficiency, but lack of incentives to improve efficiency—and in some cases considerable opposition to any form of cost or medical audit or to proposed new methods of working— may be far more serious barriers to efficiency than lack of data. As Mills remarks, a most important question is what organizational pattern provides the right incentives to doctors and to other health personnel to be cost-effective and to look for ways of delivering better care at less cost. As Ferster and Tilden add, the necessary elements are motivation, supervision, and support to sustain and improve the performance of all levels of health manpower, but how to promote these elements is not well understood. It can be concluded that in many developing countries, the scope for financial (and non-monetary) rewards and penalties to health workers and managers, encouraging them to limit costs and improve productivity, is a territory yet to be explored.

VIII. Organizational behaviour

Given the multiplicity of influential groups (such as the health professions, consumer groups, political groupings, international agencies) with interests at stake in the health sectors of many countries, it would seem prudent to focus attention on their organizations, their objectives and their behaviour. Hence, economists might profitably concern themselves with finding out the answers to such crucial questions as who makes the resource allocation decisions; what are the objectives of the decision-makers; and what type of model is most appropriate both for the study of policy-making and policy implementation (Lee 1982*b*) and for health planning. For instance, Ferster and Tilden put forward the hypothesis that if manpower planning follows the 'advocate' model, only those services will be provided that the most influential consumers and/or producers demand, and that the special interests of different groups, including key political figures, encourage. Rather different outcomes might follow from other models of policy-making, and quite different policy-making and political structures will exist between and within developing countries.

Policy-making and planning is often exceedingly complicated because of the need to take account of many interdependencies and to mobilize the necessary resources at all levels. Local constraints to implementation exist, divergent views will persist, and interested parties need to be aware of each other's point of view and of the value of working together. Hence, an understanding of the issues of decentralization, of community participation, and of the necessary and sufficient conditions for plans to be implemented is called for.

IX. Project.evaluation

Prescott and Warford argue that resource allocation decisions in health have in the past been notoriously inefficient and inequitable; and these are now reflected in an emphasis on expensive urban and hospital-based curative care which is not directed at the major causes of ill-health in the majority of developing countries. But how might efficiency be measured? While at an aggregate level improvements in health care may result in improvements in health, to measure the precise linkages between inputs and outputs, that is the production function, and hence to assess the efficiency of specific health services, is far from easy in many cases. In some, however, it is comparatively straightforward: Creese considers the most efficient way of expanding the immunization programme in the light of existing coverage levels, possible combinations of fixed and mobile services of different types, and changing input prices. He is able to employ cost–effectiveness analysis to present a series of choices capable of yielding better performance from a given budget.

The central difficulty in measuring output in terms of changes in health status is that health is not homogeneous, since health interventions can produce reductions in both morbidity and mortality. So in which units should improvements in health status be counted, let alone valued, in cost–benefit studies? The lack of a common unit seriously hampers any analytical work which purports to look at different options: as Wheeler notes, a formal test of cost-effectiveness is unhelpful in choosing the preferred option if the candidates are a disease eradication project, a health centre construction programme, and a manpower training programme, since each yields substantially different forms of output. Prescott and Warford in their survey chapter are led to conclude that the issue of benefit measurement and valuation in health projects has yet to be resolved satisfactorily. On a more optimistic note, it is clear from Wheeler's chapter that considerable scope does exist to improve health planning methodologies by incorporating simple economic evaluation techniques as a routine planning procedure early on in the planning process.

X. Health policy, equity, and social justice

Whose values should count in health policy-making and planning? The issues surrounding valuation in health and health care are fraught with difficulties. Given that decisions about priorities are made in the health sector, then judgements are explicitly or implicitly made on the value of life itself. But what is an appropriate source of values? Should the values of the doctor or the medical administrator be accepted, or the views of the consumer or the community? While it is convenient to assume that 'society' can express preferences and desires, who speaks for society at the national or at the local level? The benefits of socioeconomic development are often distributed in ways that are not considered by everyone to be equitable, and the character and distribution of health needs and the services made available to meet them may not correspond at all closely.

Equity considerations are often given considerable weight in health policy documents in many countries, but it cannot be assumed that national health and welfare policies will necessarily be equitable once implemented. As Prescott and Warford point out, if distributional objectives are important, then analyses of the distribution of expenditure by beneficiaries in different income classes, or simply by region, should assist policy-makers. Lee emphasizes that it is necessary to disentangle issues of rich and poor from those of geographical location, since the health facilities in urban areas may be accessible only to the urban elite. When inequalities are of major significance, it is likely to be necessary also to disentangle issues of income insufficiency from issues of power. Westcott suggests that if it is accepted that in developing countries the main nutritional objective is to reduce malnutrition, since those who suffer from malnutrition are likely to be worst off financially, and since the distribution of food tends also to correspond to the distribution of power in a country, one may be sceptical about the possibility of changing one without the other. What values economists or others should use in their analyses is debatable: the definition of 'justice' adopted in a country will reflect those whose perspectives and perceptions are most influential in the policy-making process. Economists must determine whether or not they are able to work within these parameters.

Political constraints

All the contributors to this volume have indicated not only the conceptual and methodological problems of relating economics to the health sector but also, with varying degrees of frankness, the institutional and political constraints which can influence whether or not economic analyses affect policies and actions. These constraints do not negate the contribution that economics can make, but they do none the less affect the actual interface between economics, health care, and health itself.

One problem stems from a common belief, mistaken or otherwise, that economics—like other theoretical disciplines—does not offer much that is relevant to policy formulation and to its implementation by managers. Economic principles are seen as either too limited and simplistic (for instance only interested in questions of money) or too abstract and remote from the real-life world of politics, power, value conflicts, bargaining, and institutional realities (WHO 1975). The lesson to be learned, so far as economic analysis is concerned, is that adequate consideration must be given to political realities and administrative feasibilities. Every decision taken in the light of an economic assessment of the issue is also one taken in the light of political constraints and value premises.

Decisions often called 'political' in a derogatory sense may in reality be responses to societal values and goals (White, Anderson, Kalimo, Kleczkowski, Purola, and Vukmanovic 1977). Decisions will reflect the shared values of a particular community if the interests of all members of the community are taken into account in both the determination of its health goals and the priorities for their attainment; the health goals of a society can be established in a similar way. But in each community and between communities there is potential for conflict: for instance, over whether the satisfaction of local needs by local means or the achievement of national uniformity of standards, policies, and approaches should be paramount. Superimposed on the inter-community and centre–periphery tussle are professional interests which, with varying degrees of success, will exert pressure to influence policies and priorities. It is only to be expected, therefore, that at least some of the barriers to the application of health economics will have their roots in the structure and decision-making processes that exist in each country. The health sector contains within it various groups with different values, and differing degrees of financial, organizational and professional autonomy. All these interest groups cannot be expected to view present and possible future situations in the same way: a conflict of interests and values, whether implicit or explicit, is only to be expected. If there is no assured consensus on values or on the objectives of health policy, this affects the role of health economists and the application of economics.

There is clearly no 'scientific' or 'value free' way of determining the allocation of resources to and within the health sector, and economists are not known for their ability to express a united view. But it would be foolish to deny the possibility that some ways are likely to be better than others. Health economics does not claim to guarantee a desired future: it is, at best, a way of exploring the possibility and desirability of various futures. How that exploration is conducted depends on the people involved as much as on the strengths of the discipline of economics.

Governments of developing countries may wish to use the health sector to help mobilize the people, to promote national integration, or to achieve a political consensus (Lee and Mills 1982). It may, in consequence, be a myth to believe that governments allocate resources to the health sector solely in order to improve the health of their populations, and even more of a myth to believe that governments are universally committed—above all else—to health improvement (England 1978). Governments will have to trade-off objectives against each other in the light of resource availability. Where health is given low priority and there is no political will for change, perhaps because the government represents the more powerful and more healthy rather than the less powerful and less healthy, then the WHO goal of health for all by the year 2000 is unlikely to be attained.

Not all decisions, of course, will be determined by vested interests. Conflict will arise only when the appropriateness of a 'technical' solution to the needs or demands of the population runs counter to the value system of those who influence policy. Yet no piece of economic analysis can be entirely shielded from political considerations. As Abel-Smith (1976) noted:

A powerful politician may have promised to secure a hospital for his constituency and he is likely to get it. Any theoretical distributional aim may be modified by short-term political pressures. These are the realities of life in any society (p. 180).

Economists should beware of letting decision-makers believe that economics has the answers to all their problems: it can help them explore and perhaps resolve some—it is not a panacea. Moreover, the quest for the most cost-effective and least-cost ways of improving health will inevitably challenge a number of government health policies and conventional patterns of thinking about health and medical care, as well as questioning the roles and functions and perhaps threatening the incomes of some existing forms of health personnel. Understandably, there may be a reluctance to face up to or implement the stark choices made explicit through economic analysis. If that is so, the principles and techniques of health economics can be of most help only to those who really desire to effect change. The rationale for using health economics and employing health economists is to detail the alternatives so that the issues involved and the choices made are clearly understood (Mooney, Russell, and Weir 1979). Choice remains the critical issue. While health economists and economics can show the way (or more often, a number of ways), governments, politicians, doctors, administrators, can choose to follow other routes. That is *their* choice.

Future strategies

The growth in the health economics literature, the increasing number of health economists working in developing countries, the growing interest amongst health workers in health economics, and the attention paid by international agencies to economic and related questions about the health sector, all bear testimony to the assistance health economics can provide in elucidating health issues. At the same time, given the size and importance of health sectors, it is still surprising that comparatively few economists have interested themselves in the health field. That picture is slowly changing but it is perhaps worth reflecting on the likely major contributory factors for this lack of numbers. These factors affect both demand and supply, though the relative importance of each is not clear.

In any analysis of the labour market for health economists, the question arises of whether a demand exists, and if so how it is being met. For reasons advanced in the previous section, it may be that policy-makers and professional groups found it convenient to avoid the painful task of improving efficiency and questioning resource allocation procedures; the political costs were perhaps too great. Conversely, policy-makers and professional groups may simply be unaware of what economics can offer; or they may be well aware of the potential contribution economics and health economists can make, but conscious that to date few economists have interested themselves in their particular problems and policies.

This latter observation suggests that evidence of the failure of economists to look at the health sector might reflect either insufficient numbers or their attitudes to themselves, to their role, and to their training. In many developing countries, economists are in short supply and the political process may give priority to economic problems as opposed to social issues, and may subordinate social goals to economic objectives. Health sector policies may be subservient to the management of the economy and economists will be concentrated where they are believed to be of most use. This subordination of social goals to economic objectives is sustained by the deeply entrenched view that social progress is a recipient and not a determinant of economic growth. It is then hardly surprising to see economists spending their time and energies on priorities consistent with those reflected in their societies generally and in their educational institutions in particular.

Economists may also feel that a certain 'mystique' exists about medicine and health care, and that barriers to entry exist in the form of a dominant medical ideology. In addition, difficulties abound in developing a model or models of the health sector, in defining health, in understanding the technology and vocabulary, and in measuring outputs. In contrast, there exists a much better established theoretical foundation and conceptual underpinning to macroeconomics and to the micro issues of the productive and financial sectors. Part of the problem also rests in the comparative richness of data about the economic sector and the relative paucity of information about many socio-economic and health-related indicators. When these various factors are brought together, they may appear insurmountable to a budding health economist who must demonstrate his professional competence to his fellow economists in other 'trades' if he is to be considered as a respected and respectable practitioner of the art of economics. In short, such considerations may account for the present underdevelopment of health economics and for the poor supply of health economists in the developing world.

One key to overcoming some of these deficiencies may lie in presenting health economics as a challenge. Increasing numbers of economists in the developed world are turning to health, recognizing that considerable scope exists for drawing on the body of economic knowledge and reforming and developing it to make it more appropriate to the health sector. It may also be necessary to convince other economists and recruits to economics that the problems which the health sector presents are, in principle, similar to those presented in both the public and private sectors. This is not to deny the existence of a combination of characteristics which are distinctive to health, but rather to argue that by studying this sector, theories may be developed which can be profitably applied to other areas of contemporary economic activity, and which add to the corpus of economic theory and techniques.

From what has already been stated, it is clear that many more professionally trained economists could and should, where they are available, be attracted into the health sector. University departments of economics need to be made more aware of the potential that exists for the application of economics, and to encourage their faculty staff, postgraduate and undergraduate students to be more knowledgeable about the present state of the art and the potential yet to be realized. Likewise, schools of public health and of medicine in developing countries could encourage the employment and training of their own faculty and graduates in the principles and techniques of economic analysis. The health sector itself and its key policy-makers and managers also need to provide greater opportunities for economists to enter the field. Clearly this end can be achieved in a number of ways and it is up to each country to decide how best it can be done. Their actions will affect the employment opportunities for those versed in health economics, and thus the provision of undergraduate and postgraduate courses.

A basic question remains to be tackled: how and where the capabilities of economists should be deployed. In order to maximize their impact on policy matters and the management of resources, some will need to work within the health sector, including in government ministries. The economist's conceptual framework is sufficiently adaptable to contribute to analysis of both strategic and operational issues, and since decision-making in the health sector takes place at different levels and involves various groups, there is no single level or group at which health economics should be aimed.

In addition to those working in the health sector, there should be economists who develop the discipline of health economics by producing teaching material relevant to the health problems of their own countries and methodologies suitable for the conduct of case studies, and by conducting research into the economics of health. The table that appears in this chapter could provide a framework for developing a research programme and a teaching curriculum in health economics. But in what kind of unit should such activities be based? Much will depend upon local circumstances and the enthusiasm and commitment of individuals. Whatever academic base is selected (economics, development studies, public health, schools of medicine), and whatever the sources of funds (government, health sector, external assistance) the unit should encourage the development of the discipline of health economics by the recruitment/ encouragement/training of local people; by modifying and adapting economic thinking to local circumstances; by performing a large part of the teaching role; and by acting as a training base for economists interested in a career in the health sector. Finally, the unit should above all be seen as a source of expert advice to which policy-makers and managers can turn.

Whether the unit is made up only of economists or of other disciplines as well (such as other social sciences and epidemiology), it should actively link with those disciplines and professions interested in policy analysis and health services research. Health economists need to be aware of the disciplinary background, approach and potential contribution of other 'team' members; the economist needs to be as willing to learn from other disciplines and to interact with other groups as he expects them to be receptive to his own ideas, theories, and models.

The nature of the relationship between economists and health officials would be further enhanced if those working in the health sector, and especially in government health services, were more familiar with the principles and techniques of health economics. This will be vital in countries where even general economists are scarce, and can anyway be helpful in ensuring that there are a number of people in the health sector who appreciate the assistance a basic knowledge of health economics can give them. Mechanisms therefore need to be established to introduce economic reasoning into such areas as the finance sections of health ministries, and to develop courses and seminars for key national/regional/state officials in applied health economics.

Countries could be faced with the dilemma of whether to invest limited resources in developing expertise in one or a few specialist units, to spread those resources to all medical schools, for example, or to concentrate on reaching health personnel and policy-makers. Such a dilemma need not exist if part of the accepted role of any health economics or health research unit is to develop a knowledge of health economics in those working in the health sector. Indeed, the latter objective is unlikely to be achieved without the manpower resources available in an academic or research unit.

What role should health economists themselves take in working with personnel in the health sector? The discussion so far has neglected the way in which health economists see their role, and the way in which they would like their role to be perceived. Economists can in general take either an 'active' or a 'passive' role in policy-making and management. The activist seeks to have some direct influence on policy; at the other end of the spectrum 'passivity' entails no demand for direct influence and advocacy is limited to the transmission of information, rather than the determination of policy. Engleman (1980), for instance, has argued that economists, if they attempt to separate fact and value, try to distance themselves from *decision-making* while wanting close involvement in the *decision-making process*. This, he argues, is expecting too much and is likely to lead to economists being regarded as remote from power politics and value conflicts, and operating on altogether too abstract a plane. Indeed, he appears to chastise those economists who believe that if they dare to permit their values to intrude into policy questions they will effectively negate whatever contribution they might otherwise make. Akehurst (1981) puts the opposing argument that once an economist opts for and advocates a particular policy on the basis of both analysis and his own value judgement, he ceases to act as an economist. Indeed, he argues that to mingle analysis with advocacy might lead the economist to be listened to less rather than more: the economist's attempts to keep his own values separate in no way disqualifies him from being involved in making recommendations. The determination of which 'type' of role is evident in practice appears to rest with those employing the health economist, who must decide what type of economist they want.

Summary and conclusion

This book began by arguing the relevance of economic theory to the problems of health and health care in developing countries. Some of the ways in which it is relevant, both in describing what is happening and why and in suggesting what can be done, have been the subject of further analysis in subsequent chapters. These chapters have demonstrated just how wide is the scope for sustained work in applying the concepts and skills of economics to the health sector. Any limits to what might be profitably undertaken, either in developing theory or in its application, are unlikely to be reached in the foreseeable future.

In the unchanging or worsening financial climate of many developing countries, it has been suggested that it is much easier for economists to be involved; for their role to be acknowledged and welcomed; and for the ideas of health economics to be recognized as highly relevant to policy determination and management. At the same time, health economics cannot be separated from other disciplines if realistic health policies are to be devised, implemented, and evaluated. The economist must combine with disciplines such as community medicine, epidemiology, statistics, engineering, sociology, and it will be their joint endeavours that will suggest least-cost, economically viable, politically acceptable, and culturally appropriate policies for health services and health.

In the future economists will increasingly be involved in the process of health policy development, so this book has tried to convey what they can and cannot bring to the process as *economists*; and likewise, what *economics* can and cannot do. Political and institutional constraints must be taken into account, though few economists are likely to be ignorant of the potential and the limitations of their theories and of the extent of their influence when it comes to final decisions about choices, priorities, and policies.

It is, none the less, important to conclude by stating that many alternative courses of action are available in the health sector and that choices have to be made. Economics is basically an attitude of mind—or an approach inculcated by training—to think about choices, alternatives, and preferences. In the final analysis, planners should be able to demonstrate that the health policies being promoted within a country are likely to result in greater benefit than could be obtained by using the same resources differently. Economists must respond to this challenge: this volume is one such response by a group of interested economists, all of whom are investing a good deal of time and energy in exploring the interface between economics, health services, and health in developing countries, and in encouraging others to do likewise.

REFERENCES

Abel-Smith, B. (1976). *Value for money in health services.* Heinemann, London.
Akehurst, R. L. (1981). Health economists and the NHS: a comment. *Community Med.* 3, 149–53.
England, R. (1978). More myths in international health planning. *Am. J. Publ. Hlth* 68, 153–9.
Engleman, S. R. (1980). Health economics, health economists and the NHS. *Community Med.* 2, 126–34.
Lee, K. (1982a). Public expenditure, health services and health. In *Public expenditure and social policy* (ed. A. Walker) pp. 73–90. Heinemann, London.
— (1982b). The economics of decision-making in the social services. *Int. J. Soc. Econ.* 9, 50–65.
— and Mills, A. (1982). *Policy-making and planning in the health sector.* Croom Helm, London.
Mooney, G. H., Russell, E. M., and Weir, R. D. (1979). *Choices for health care.* Macmillan, London.
White, K. L., Anderson, D. O., Kalimo, E., Kleczkowski, B. M., Purola, T., and Vukmanovic, C. (1977). Health services: concepts and information for national planning and management. *Publ. Hlth Pap. WHO* 67.
WHO (World Health Organization) (1975). Health economics. *Publ. Hlth Pap. WHO* 64.

Authors' note

This final chapter has drawn upon both the authors' own experience and knowledge of developing countries and upon the discussions with the other contributors to this volume. Some of the points raised in this chapter first appeared in a paper entitled: 'Health care in the developing world: the role of economists and economics', which was presented at an International Interdisciplinary Workshop on *Health and development in Africa* in Bayreuth, Federal Republic of Germany, May 1982. The authors wish to acknowledge the help they have received in clarifying the ideas expressed in this chapter; any remaining errors are, of course, their own.

Index

volunteers 109, 110, 121
  see also workers, health
comprehensive model 118-19
congenital conditions 28
consumption
  demand, 39
  expenditure 24, 28
  food, influences on 171-3;
  health as 93
  of health services, determinants of 36-8
co-operatives
  health insurance in 80, 82
  source of finance for health care 96
Coovadia, H. H. 169
Correa, H. 182
cost
  containment 78, 79, 82, 129, 222
  of disease 12, 15
  of disease control 15
  escalation 43, 73, 77-8
  functions 17
  of health services 16, 38
  marginal 106-7, 129, 140, 179
  of primary health care 9, 18, 82, 95-6,
    99-100, 111-12
  recurrent 129-31, 194
  of reducing infant and child mortality 40
  social 179-80, 210
  unit 129
  see also cost-benefit analysis; cost-
    effectiveness analysis; opportunity
    cost
cost-benefit analysis
  of immunization 151-5
  of nutrition programmes 182-4, 186-7
  shadow pricing in 139-40, 152-3, 155
  techniques 135-8, 147, 213
  treatment of uncertainty 138-9
cost-effectiveness analysis
  of alternative approaches 102-4, 106-7,
    204, 221
  in manpower planning 123
  of nutrition programmes 180-2
  shadow pricing in 139-40, 163-4
  techniques 131-5, 148, 202, 213
  of training methods 117
  treatment of uncertainty 138-9
  of ways of reducing infant mortality
    155-62
  within immunization programmes 162-4
cost-sharing 72, 81, 85
co-trimoxazole 104
country health programming 14, 48, 159,
  204-6
Cox, P. 105
Cravioto, J. 170, 185
Creese, A. 106, 163
Cullis, J. G. 74
Culyer, A. J. 10, 11, 13, 64, 134, 137

Cummins, G. 183
Cumper, G. 14, 15, 29, 35, 48, 82
curative medicine 35, 45, 49, 82, 91, 120,
  141, 146
customs duties 65
Cvejtanovic, B. 152

DAIS 94-5
Daly, J. A. 50
Dasgupta, P. S. 137, 139, 180
data banks 33
Day, S. R. 132
DDT 29, 39, 40
death rates 6, 92; *see also* child mortality
  rate; infant mortality rate
debility 8, 12
decentralization 119
deductibles 72, 98
Deering J. A. 47
degenerative conditions 28, 30
de la Grandville, O. 50
demand
  consumer 41
  definition of 70, 211
  determinants of 70-1, 72, 73, 74, 220-1
  effect of insurance on 78
  elasticity 70-1, 141, 175, 181
  functions 17, 138, 175-6
  for health care 64, 121, 195
  for primary health care 96, 100-1, 111
  for private health insurance 67-8
Denmark, national health service in 66
dentists, sensitivity to price 37
Department of Health and Social Security
  (DHSS) 149
developed countries
  economic indicators of 1, 27
  epidemiology of 91
  social and cultural characteristics 27
developing countries 1
  classification of 3
  economic indicators of 3-6, 126
  economists in 11
  health indicators of 6-9
  health economics in 12, 13-15
  medical insurance in 65
development theory 23-5, 93
  and economic models 191-5, 196-7
de Vries, J. L. 132
diagnostic services 45
diarrhoeal diseases 8, 28
diet
  effect on health 29
  and of shift to cash production 31
Dievler, A. 132
diphtheria 148, 149, 159
disability 8, 12, 31, 45, 134, 137
discount rate 155
discriminant analysis 33

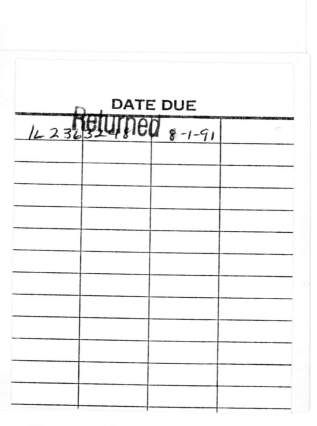